The Se\

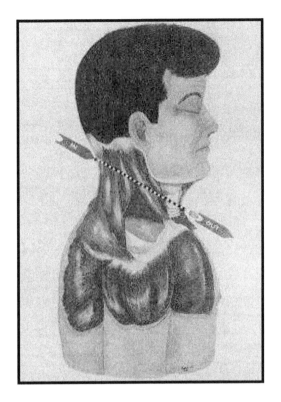

of the Medical Evidence
and the Shot That Killed JFK
By
Patrick Harris, Ph.D.

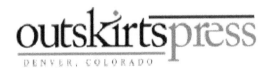

outskirtspress

DENVER, COLORADO

On the Preceding Page: Redrawn version of Warren Commission Exhibit 385 showing a bullet passing through the President at 29 degrees, the unadjusted angle of declination from the westernmost sixth floor window of the Texas School Book Depository at Zapruder Frame 227. The entrance point corresponds to the entrance wound at the base of the President's skull, as determined at autopsy and by the Warren Commission, and the exit point corresponds to the exit wound found in the President's neck. This shot killed the President five seconds before the so-called "head shot".

Dedicated To
Anna Brennan

TABLE OF CONTENTS

(handwritten margin notes:) yes; yes; NO

(handwritten next to chapter 14:) 14 Shots 13 Hits

(handwritten notes at bottom:)
Various
1 DalTex —
2 Mac Wallace
3 Corsicans (2)
4 County Records Bldg (LEO)
5 Perogilla (2)
6 another (LEO)

INTRODUCTION

It is difficult for those born after 1960 to imagine what kind of a nation America was, and ultimately became, in 1963. America had defeated the Axis powers on two fronts only eighteen years prior, ushering in the atomic age with unimagined force. By 1963 America was launching men into space, with a commitment to put a man on the moon by the end of the decade. America was by far the world leader in technology and diplomacy, and had just stared down the Soviet menace in Cuba.

Presiding over the American juggernaut was a man of incredible wit and charm, whose level of dynamism and charisma had never been seen before in the White House. John F. Kennedy's handsome good looks and vital bearing cemented America's standing as a world leader, and his beautiful and elegant wife was his perfect complement as first lady.

America was a nation on the move, a confident land of infinite promise, of unlimited possibilities. America was on top of the world, and the Kennedys were the toast of America.

And suddenly it all came crashing down in a hail of bullets in Dallas. In its aftermath America and the rest of the world were stunned into days of mourning, incredulous that a man so admired had been taken so horribly in the blink of an eye. It was an event that still resonates in America to this day.

The essential facts of the crime are well known: while riding through Dallas on November 22, 1963, the President was shot and then transported to a nearby hospital, where he died. His body was brought back to Washington for an autopsy. He was subsequently mourned for two days in a closed casket at the U.S. Capitol, and was then buried after a funeral that included many world leaders. The new President, Lyndon Johnson, appointed a Commission to examine the matter. The Commission reported back that President Kennedy was killed by a lone sniper with World Communist sympathies, who had previously defected to the Soviet Union, and who had

Bed Time Story

1

been recently spotted at the Soviet and Cuban embassies in Mexico. The sniper, Lee Harvey Oswald, was then shot and killed by local strip club operator Jack Ruby, allegedly because Ruby wanted to spare Jacqueline Kennedy the grief of having to testify at Oswald's trial.

From there the facts, fiction, and fantasy fairy-tale thinking diverge astronomically in all directions while attempting to explain who killed the President, how it was accomplished, and why it was done. The debate reaches into the very heart and soul of America in a way that is unique in American history.

President Kennedy was immensely popular at the time of his death, but underneath the surface of polite manners there were deep reservoirs of vitriolic hate for the President. After Fidel Castro seized control of Cuba and prevailed at the Bay of Pigs in 1961, anti-Castro Cubans felt abandoned and betrayed by the President. The Mafia thought he was an obstacle to their reclaiming Havana as their own, and objected to Robert Kennedy's crackdown on organized crime, particularly since they believed they had helped Kennedy to achieve the Presidency. Mafia kingpin Carlos Marcello in particular felt an intense hatred for the Kennedys after they unceremoniously deported him to Guatemala, leaving him to fend for himself far from civilization. The top men at the CIA were fired by the President after the Bay of Pigs debacle, and many in the CIA feared losing their jobs to the President's threat to reorganize or eliminate the agency. Vice President Lyndon Johnson and FBI Director J. Edgar Hoover were both destined to lose their jobs and power with a continued Kennedy Presidency, and Johnson was headed for a jail cell.

America may have loved the President, but there were those with every incentive to kill him.

CHAPTER 1

THE OFFICIAL VERSIONS I:
THE WARREN COMMISSION

BedTime Stary

The official version of the assassination is comprised of three federal judicial inquiries: the Warren Commission (1963 – 1964), the Clark Panel (1968 - 1969), and the House Select Committee on Assassinations (1976 – 1979), as well as the memoranda and formal pronouncements of federal agencies such as the FBI, CIA, and the Department of Justice.

Two additional federal panels, The President's Commission on CIA Activities within the United States (1975), chaired by Vice President Nelson Rockefeller, and the Senate Select Committee to Study Governmental Operations with Respect to Intelligence Activities (1976), chaired by Senator Frank Church, tangentially examined the potential role of the CIA in the President's assassination. Both found no evidence of CIA involvement.

The findings of all three Kennedy assassination inquiries differ in several respects, particularly with regard to the location of the President's wounds, in what appears to have been a staged charade of media manipulation and manufactured truth. Even within the Warren Commission Report itself one of the President's wounds inexplicably migrates from its established location on the autopsy face sheet and clothing bullet holes to a location five inches away in the Commission's published exhibits.

Shortly after the assassination President Lyndon Johnson spoke with FBI Director J. Edgar Hoover about the need to create a federal panel to circumvent congressional inquiries and rely solely on Hoover's version of events:

Hoover: I've seen the reports on the Senate investigating committee they've been talking about.

Johnson: Well we think if we don't have…I want to get by just with your file and your report.

Hoover: I think it would be very, very bad to have a rash of investigations on this thing.

Johnson: Well the only way we can stop 'em is probably to appoint a high level one to evaluate your report.

Hoover: Yes.

Johnson: And put somebody that's pretty good on it from, that I can select out of the government, and tell the House and Senate not to go ahead with an investigation.

Hoover: Yes.

Johnson: 'Cause we get up there and get a bunch of television going, and I thought it'd be bad.

Hoover: It'd be a three-ring circus. [1] *True*

On November 29, 1963 Lyndon Johnson signed an executive order creating the President's Commission on the Assassination of President Kennedy, commonly known as the Warren Commission, after its chairman, Chief Justice of the Supreme Court Earl Warren.

The Commission completed its work on September 24, 1964. The Commission's report was made available to the public in two stages: the principal report was released on September 27, 1964, and the 26 volumes of supporting testimony and exhibits followed several months later, after the November 1964 presidential election.

The Commission described its mandate and performance in lofty and glowing terms:

"By his order of November 29 establishing the Commission, President Johnson sought to avoid parallel investigations and to concentrate

4

base of the back of the neck. The autopsy report stated the cause of death as 'Gunshot wound, head,' and the bullets which struck the President were described as having been fired 'from a point behind and somewhat above the level of the deceased.'

At the scene of the shooting, there was evident confusion at the outset concerning the point of origin of the shots. Witnesses differed in their accounts of the direction from which the sound of the shots emanated. Within a few minutes, however, attention centered on the Texas School Book Depository Building as the source of the shots...[5]

Several eyewitnesses in front of the building reported that they saw a rifle being fired from the southeast corner window on the sixth floor of the Texas School Book Depository. One eyewitness, Howard L. Brennan, had been watching the parade from a point on Elm Street directly opposite and facing the building. He promptly told a policeman that he had seen a slender man, about 5 feet 10 inches, in his early thirties, take deliberate aim from the sixth-floor corner window and fire a rifle in the direction of the President's car." [6]

Mac Wallace

An employee of the School Book Depository, Lee Harvey Oswald, soon became a focus of the search.

"Approximately 7 minutes later, at about 12:40 p.m., Oswald boarded a bus at a point on Elm Street seven short blocks east of the Depository Building. The bus was traveling west toward the very building from which Oswald had come. Its route lay through the Oak Cliff section in southwest Dallas, where it would pass seven blocks east of the roominghouse in which Oswald was living, at 1026 North Beckley Avenue. On the bus was Mrs. Mary Bledsoe, one of Oswald's former landladies who immediately recognized him. Oswald stayed on the bus approximately 3 or 4 minutes, during which time it proceeded only two blocks because of the traffic jam created by the motorcade and the assassination. Oswald then left the bus.

7

A few minutes later he entered a vacant taxi four blocks away and asked the driver to take him to a point on North Beckley Avenue several blocks beyond his roominghouse. The trip required 5 or 6 minutes. At about 1 p.m. Oswald arrived at the roominghouse. The housekeeper, Mrs. Earlene Roberts, was surprised to see Oswald at midday and remarked to him that he seemed to be in quite a hurry. He made no reply. A few minutes later Oswald emerged from his room zipping up his jacket and rushed out of the house.

Approximately 14 minutes later, and just 45 minutes after the assassination, another violent shooting occurred in Dallas. The victim was Patrolman J.D. Tippit of the Dallas police, an officer with a good record during his more than 11 years with the police force. He was shot near the intersection of 10th Street and Patton Avenue, about nine-tenths of a mile from Oswald's roominghouse...[7]

never promoted + GED

At approximately 1:15 p.m., Tippit was driving slowly in an easterly direction on East 10th Street in Oak Cliff. About 100 feet past the intersection of 10th Street and Patton Avenue, Tippit pulled up alongside a man walking in the same direction. The man met the general description of the suspect wanted in connection with the assassination. He walked over to Tippit's car, rested his arms on the door on the right-hand side of the car, and apparently exchanged words with Tippit through the window. Tippit opened the door on the left side and started to walk around the front of his car. As he reached the front wheel on the driver's side, the man on the sidewalk drew a revolver and fired several shots in rapid succession, hitting Tippit four times and killing him instantly. An automobile repairman, Domingo Benavides, heard the shots and stopped his pickup truck on the opposite side of the street about 25 feet in front of Tippit's car. He observed the gunman start back toward Patton Avenue, removing the empty cartridge cases from the gun as he went...[8]

Shortly before 1 p.m. Capt. J. Will Fritz, chief of the homicide and robbery bureau of the Dallas Police Department, arrived to take charge of the investigation. Searching the sixth floor, Deputy Sheriff Luke Mooney noticed a pile of cartons in the southeast corner. He squeezed through the boxes and realized immediately that he had discovered the point from which the shots had been fired. On the floor were three empty cartridge cases. A carton had apparently been placed on the floor at the side of the window so that a person sitting on the carton could look down Elm Street toward the overpass and scarcely be noticed from the outside. Between this carton and the half-open window were three additional cartons arranged at such an angle that a rifle resting on the top carton would be aimed directly at the motorcade as it moved away from the building. The high stack of boxes, which first attracted Mooney's attention, effectively screened a person at the window from the view of anyone else on the floor.

Mooney's discovery intensified the search for additional evidence on the sixth floor, and at 1:22 p.m., approximately 10 minutes after the cartridge cases were found, Deputy Sheriff Eugene Boone turned his flashlight in the direction of two rows of boxes in the northwest corner near the staircase. Stuffed between the two rows was a bolt-action rifle with a telescopic sight. The rifle was not touched until it could be photographed. When Lt. J.C. Day of the police identification bureau decided that the wooden stock and the metal knob at the end of the bolt contained no prints, he held the rifle by the stock while Captain Fritz ejected a live shell by operating the bolt. Lieutenant Day promptly noted that stamped on the rifle itself was the serial number 'C2766' as well as the markings '1940' 'MADE ITALY' and 'CAL 6.5.' The rifle was about 40 inches long and when disassembled it could fit into a handmade paper sack which, after the assassination, was found in the southeast corner of the building within a few feet of the cartridge cases..." [9]

The Commission spared no effort in describing Oswald as a psychologically troubled youth, and later, as an ardent Communist:

MARXIST

"In January 1944, when Lee was 4, he was taken out of the orphanage, and shortly thereafter his mother moved with him to Dallas, Tex., where the older boys joined them at the end of the school year. In May of 1945 Marguerite Oswald married her third husband, Edwin A. Ekdahl. While the two older boys attended a military boarding school, Lee lived at home and developed a warm attachment to Ekdahl, occasionally accompanying his mother and stepfather on business trips around the country. Lee started school in Benbrook, Tex., but in the fall of 1946, after a separation from Ekdahl, Marguerite Oswald reentered Lee in the first grade in Covington, La. In January 1947, while Lee was still in the first grade, the family moved to Fort Worth, Tex., as the result of an attempted reconciliation between Ekdahl and Lee's mother. A year and a half later, before Lee was 9, his mother was divorced from her third husband as the result of a divorce action instituted by Ekdahl. Lee's school record during the next 5 ½ years in Fort Worth was average, although generally it grew poorer each year. The comments of teachers and others who knew him at that time do not reveal any unusual personality traits or characteristics.

Another change for Lee Oswald occurred in August 1952, a few months after he completed the sixth grade. Marguerite Oswald and her 12-year-old son moved to New York City where Marguerite's oldest son, John Pic, was stationed with the Coast Guard. The ensuing year and one-half in New York was marked by Lee's refusals to attend school and by emotional and psychological problems of a seemingly serious nature. Because he had become a chronic school truant, Lee underwent psychiatric study at Youth House, an institution in New York for juveniles who have had truancy problems or difficulties with the law, and who appear to require psychiatric observation, or other types of guidance. The social worker assigned to his case described him as 'seriously detached' and 'withdrawn' and noted 'a rather pleasant, appealing quality about this emotionally starved, affectionless youngster.' Lee expressed the feeling to the social worker that his mother did not care for him and regarded him as a burden. He experienced fantasies about being all powerful and hurting people, but during his stay at Youth House he was apparently not a behavior problem. He appeared withdrawn and evasive, a boy who preferred to spend his time alone, reading and watching television. His tests indicated that he was above average in intelligence for his age group. The chief psychiatrist of Youth House diagnosed Lee's problem as a 'personality pattern disturbance with schizoid features and passive-aggressive tendencies.' He concluded that the boy was 'an emotionally, quite disturbed youngster' and recommended psychiatric treatment.

In May 1953, after having been at Youth House for 3 weeks, Lee Oswald returned to school where his attendance and grades temporarily improved. By the following fall, however, the probation officer reported that virtually every teacher complained about the boy's behavior. His mother insisted that he did not need psychiatric assistance. Although there was apparently some improvement in Lee's behavior during the next few months, the court recommended further treatment. In January 1954, while Lee's case was still pending, Marguerite and Lee left for New Orleans, the city of Lee's birth." [10]

After turning 16 Oswald left school.

"After leaving school Lee worked the next 10 months at several jobs in New Orleans as an office messenger or clerk. It was during this period that he started to read communist literature. Occasionally, in conversations with others, he praised communism and expressed to his fellow employees a desire to join the Communist Party. At about this time, when he was not yet 17, he wrote to the Socialist Party of America, professing his belief in Marxism.

Another move followed in July 1956 when Lee and his mother returned to Fort Worth. He reentered high school but again dropped out after a few weeks and enlisted in the Marine Corps on October 24, 1956, 6 days after his 17th birthday. On December 21, 1956, during boot camp in San Diego, Oswald fired a score of 212 for record with the M-1 rifle – 2 points over the minimum for a rating of 'sharpshooter' on a marksman / sharpshooter / expert scale. After his basic training, Oswald received training in aviation fundamentals and then in radar scanning.

Most people who knew Oswald in the Marines described him as a 'loner' who resented the exercise of authority by others. He spent much of his free time reading. He was court-martialed once for possessing an unregistered privately owned weapon and, on another occasion, for using provocative language to a noncommissioned officer. He was, however, generally able to comply with Marine discipline, even though his experiences in the Marine Corps did not live up to his expectations.

Oswald served 15 months overseas until November 1958, most of it in Japan. During his final year in the Marine Corps he was stationed for the most part in Santa Ana, Calif., where he showed a marked interest in the Soviet Union and sometimes expressed politically radical views with dogmatic conviction. Oswald again fired the M-1 rifle for record on May 6, 1959, and this time he shot a score of 191 on a shorter course than before, only 1 point over the minimum required to be a 'marksman'. According to one of his fellow marines, Oswald was not particularly interested in his rifle performance, and his unit was not expected to exhibit the usual rifle proficiency. During this period he expressed strong admiration for Fidel Castro and an interest in joining the Cuban army." [11]

Oswald completed his service with the Marines in September 1959. A few weeks later he defected to the Soviet Union, where he met and married his wife, Marina Prusakova, and had a child. He returned to the United States in June 1962, along with his wife and infant. [12]

"For a few weeks Oswald, his wife and child lived with Oswald's brother Robert. After a similar stay with Oswald's mother, they moved into their own apartment in early August. Oswald obtained a job on July 16 as a sheet metal worker. During this period in Fort Worth, Oswald was interviewed twice by agents of the FBI. The report of the first interview, which occurred on June 26, described him as arrogant and unwilling to discuss the reasons why he had gone to the Soviet Union. Oswald denied that he was involved in Soviet intelligence activities and promised to advise the FBI if Soviet representatives ever communicated with him. He was interviewed again on August 16, when he displayed a less belligerent attitude and once again agreed to inform the FBI of any attempt to enlist him in intelligence activities. PAID INFORMANT $200 a month FBI /CIA/

In early October 1962 Oswald quit his job at the sheet metal plant and moved to Dallas. While living in Fort Worth the Oswalds had been introduced to a group of Russian-speaking people in the Dallas-Fort Worth area. Many of them assisted the Oswalds by providing small amounts of food, clothing, and household items. Oswald himself was disliked by almost all of this group whose help to the family was prompted primarily by sympathy for Marina Oswald and the child. Despite the fact that he had left the Soviet Union, disillusioned with its Government, Oswald seemed more firmly committed than ever to his concepts of Marxism. He showed disdain for democracy, capitalism, and American society in general. He was highly critical of the Russian-speaking group because they seemed devoted to American concepts of democracy and capitalism and were ambitious to improve themselves economically.

In February 1963 the Oswalds met Ruth Paine at a social gathering. Ruth Paine was temporarily separated from her husband and living with her two children in their home in Irving, Tex., a suburb of Dallas. Because of an interest in the Russian language and sympathy for Marina Oswald, who spoke no English and had little funds, Ruth Paine befriended Marina and, during the next 2 months, visited her on several occasions.

On April 6, 1963, Oswald lost his job with a photography firm. A few days later, on April 10, he attempted to kill Maj. Gen. Edwin A. Walker (Resigned, U.S. Army), using a rifle which he had ordered by mail 1 month previously under an assumed name. Marina Oswald learned of her husband's act when she confronted him with a note which he had left, giving her instructions in the event he did not return. That incident and their general economic difficulties impelled Marina Oswald to suggest that her husband leave Dallas and go to New Orleans to look for work.

Oswald left for New Orleans on April 24, 1963. Ruth Paine, who knew nothing of the Walker shooting, invited Marina Oswald and the baby to stay with her in the Paine's modest home while Oswald sought work in New Orleans. Early in May, upon receiving word from Oswald that he had found a job, Ruth Paine drove Marina Oswald and the baby to New Orleans to rejoin Oswald.

During the stay in New Orleans, Oswald formed a fictitious New Orleans Chapter of the Fair Play for Cuba Committee. He posed as secretary of this organization and represented that the president was A.J. Hidell. In reality, Hidell was a completely fictitious person created by Oswald, the organization's only member. Oswald was arrested on August 9 in connection with a scuffle which occurred while he was distributing pro-Castro leaflets. The next day, while at the police station, he was interviewed by an FBI agent after Oswald requested the police to arrange such an interview. Oswald gave the agent false information about his own background and was evasive in his replies concerning Fair Play for Cuba activities. During the next 2 weeks Oswald appeared on radio programs twice, claiming to be the spokesman for the Fair Play for Cuba Committee in New Orleans.

On July 19, 1963, Oswald lost his job as a greaser of coffee processing machinery. In September, after an exchange of correspondence with Marina Oswald, Ruth Paine drove to New Orleans and on September 23, transported Marina, the child, and the family belongings to Irving, Tex. Ruth Paine suggested that Marina Oswald, who was expecting her second child in October, live at the Paine house until after the baby was born. Oswald remained behind, ostensibly to find work either in Houston or some other city. Instead, he departed by bus for Mexico, arriving in Mexico City on September 27, where he promptly visited the Cuban and Russian Embassies. His stated objective was to obtain official permission to visit Cuba, on his way to the Soviet Union..." [13]

Oswald was refused and returned to Dallas, where:

"For 1 week he rented a room from Mrs. Bledsoe, the woman who later saw him on the bus shortly after the assassination. On October

14, 1963, he rented the Beckley Avenue room and listed his name as O.H. Lee. On the same day, at the suggestion of a neighbor, Mrs. Paine phoned the Texas School Book Depository and was told that there was a job opening. She informed Oswald who was interviewed the following day at the Depository and started to work there on October 16, 1963...[14]

...Oswald established a general pattern of weekend visits to Irving, arriving on Friday afternoon and returning to Dallas Monday morning with a fellow employee, Buell Wesley Frazier, who lived near the Paines...[15]

On Thursday, November 21, Oswald told Frazier that he would like to drive to Irving to pick up some curtain rods for an apartment in Dallas...[16]

The following morning Oswald left while his wife was still in bed feeding the baby. She did not see him leave the house, nor did Ruth Paine. On the dresser in their room he left his wedding ring which he had never done before. His wallet containing $170 was left intact in a dresser-drawer.

Oswald walked to Frazier's house about half a block away and placed a long bulky package, made out of wrapping paper and tape, into the rear seat of the car. He told Frazier that the package contained curtain rods. When they reached the Depository parking lot, Oswald walked quickly ahead. Frazier followed and saw Oswald enter the Depository Building carrying the long bulky package with him." [17]

Soon after the assassination and Officer Tippit's murder Oswald was arrested in the nearby Texas Theatre and brought to police headquarters.

— mono gram house

"At 7:10 p.m. on November 22, 1963, Lee Harvey Oswald was formally advised that he had been charged with the murder of Patrolman J.D. Tippit. Several witnesses to the Tippit slaying and to the subsequent flight of the gunman had positively identified Oswald in police lineups. While positive firearm identification evidence was

WRONG

15

not available at the time, the revolver in Oswald's possession at the time of his arrest was of a type which could have fired the shots that killed Tippit. ~ Shot by MAFIA or cockoled husband

The formal charge against Oswald for the assassination of President Kennedy was lodged shortly after 1:30 a.m., on Saturday, November 23. By 10 p.m. of the day of the assassination, the FBI had traced the rifle found on the sixth floor of the Texas School Book Depository to a mailorder house in Chicago which had purchased it from a distributor in New York. Approximately 6 hours later the Chicago firm advised that this rifle had been ordered in March 1963 by an A. Hidel for shipment to post office box 2915, in Dallas, Tex., a box rented by Oswald. Payment for the rifle was remitted by a money order signed by A. Hidell. By 6:45 p.m. on November 23, the FBI was able to advise the Dallas police that, as a result of handwriting analysis of the documents used to purchase the rifle, it had concluded that the rifle had been ordered by Lee Harvey Oswald...[18]

Efforts by the news media representatives to reconstruct the crime and promptly report details frequently led to erroneous and often conflicting reports. At the urgings of the newsmen, Chief of Police Jesse E. Curry, brought Oswald to a press conference in the police assembly room shortly after midnight of the day Oswald was arrested. The assembly room was crowded with newsmen who had come to Dallas from all over the country. They shouted questions at Oswald and flashed cameras at him. Among this group was a 52-year-old Dallas nightclub operator – Jack Ruby." [19]

mafia gun runner

Less than 36 hours later Ruby would shoot and kill Oswald in the basement of Dallas Police Headquarters.

THE CONCLUSIONS OF THE WARREN COMMISSION

Based on their review and analysis of the forensic evidence and witness testimony, the Warren Commission concluded:

1. The shots which killed President Kennedy and wounded Governor Connally were fired by Lee Harvey Oswald from the sixth floor window at the southeast corner of the Texas School Book Depository; Oswald killed Dallas Police Patrolman J.D. Tippit approximately 45 minutes after the assassination.

FALSE

2. The three used cartridge cases found near the window on the sixth floor came from the same Mannlicher-Carcano rifle that fired the nearly whole bullet found on a stretcher at Parkland Memorial Hospital and two other bullet fragments that were found in the front seat of the Presidential limousine. *the nope wrong again*

FALSE

3. The nature of the bullet wounds suffered by President Kennedy and Governor Connally and the location of the car at the time of the shots establish that the bullets were fired from above and behind the Presidential limousine. *and the side + front*

4. President Kennedy was first struck by a bullet which entered at the back of his neck and exited through the lower front portion of his neck, causing a wound that would not necessarily have been lethal; the President was struck a second time by a bullet which entered the right rear portion of his head, causing a massive and fatal wound.

FALSE

5. Governor Connally was struck by a bullet which entered on the right side of his back and traveled downward through the right side of his chest, exiting below his right nipple; this bullet then passed through his right wrist and entered his left thigh where it caused a superficial wound. *14 = 13 Shots 1 Miss*

6. The weight of evidence indicates that three shots were fired.

7. The Commission found no evidence that either Lee Harvey Oswald or Jack Ruby was part of any conspiracy, domestic or foreign, to assassinate President Kennedy; the Commission concluded that Oswald acted alone.

nope

F
/
A
L
S
e

8. The Commission discovered no relationship between Lee Harvey Oswald and Jack Ruby, nor was it been able to find any credible evidence that either knew the other; the Commission found no evidence that Jack Ruby acted with any other person in the killing of Lee Harvey Oswald.

9. The Commission found no credible evidence that Ruby, Tippit, or Oswald knew each other. [20]

False

THE PRESIDENT'S WOUNDS
AT PARKLAND MEMORIAL HOSPITAL

After the shooting the President was brought to Parkland Memorial Hospital for emergency resuscitation efforts. Warren Commission Exhibit 392 and Commission Price Exhibits 2 – 35 contain medical reports and admission notes filed by doctors, nurses and staff at the hospital. The reports concerning President Kennedy were written within a few hours of his assassination.

T
R
U
e

With regard to the President's wounds, all of the reports disclose essentially the same clinical picture: President Kennedy had a small wound in the front of his throat, and a large wound on the right side of the back of his head. Both cerebral and cerebellar tissue were protruding from the large wound, with the overlying skull and scalp missing. There is also mention of significant damage to the right side of the President's chest.

Dr. Kemp Clark, Director of Neurological Surgery, wrote:

"Two external wounds, one in the lower third of the anterior neck, the other in the occipital region of the skull, were noted. Through the head wound, blood and brain were extruding. Dr. Carrico inserted a cuffed endotracheal tube. While doing so, he noted a ragged wound of the trachea immediately below the larynx…There was a large wound in the right occipito-parietal region, from which profuse bleeding was occurring. 1500 cc. of blood were estimated on the drapes and floor of the Emergency Operating Room. There was considerable loss of scalp and bone tissue. Both cerebral and cerebellar tissue were extruding from the wound…There was a large wound beginning in the right occiput extending into the parietal region. Much of the skull appeared gone at brief examination." [21]

Dr. Marion Jenkins, Professor and Chairman of the Department of Anesthesiology, wrote:

"Doctors Charles Baxter, Malcolm Perry and Robert McClelland arrived at the same time and began a tracheostomy and started the insertion of a right chest tube, since there was also obvious tracheal and chest damage…There was a great laceration on the right side of the head (temporal and occipital), causing a great defect in the skull plate so that there was herniation and laceration of great areas of the brain, even to the extent that the cerebellum had protruded from the wound." [22]

Dr. Charles Baxter wrote:

"…temporal and occipital bones were missing…" [23]

Dr. Malcolm Perry wrote:

"…A large wound of the right posterior cranium was noted, exposing severely lacerated brain…" [24]

Dr. Charles Carrico wrote:

"…attempt to control slow oozing from cerebral and cerebellar tissue…" [25]

Nurse Patricia Hutton wrote:

"…Mr. Kennedy was bleeding profusely from a wound on the back of his head, and was lying there unresponsive…A doctor asked me to place a pressure dressing on the head wound. This was of no use, however, because of the massive opening on the back of the head..." [26]

In addition to these clinical reports, Clint Hill, the Secret Service agent seen jumping onto the back of the President's limousine, provided testimony to the Warren Commission concerning the President's condition at the hospital:

Mr. Specter: What did you observe as to President Kennedy's condition on arrival at the hospital?

Mr. Hill: The right rear portion of his head was missing. It was lying in the rear seat of the car. His brain was exposed. There was blood and bits of brain all over the entire rear portion of the car. Mrs. Kennedy was completely covered with blood. There was so much blood you could not tell if there had been any other wound or not, except for the one large gaping wound in the right rear portion of the head. [27]

All of these accounts note a large wound in the back of the President's head, with many indicating the protrusion of cerebellar tissue out of that wound.

Using the major lobes of the brain as anatomical landmarks (Figure 1-1), the attending physicians' written accounts establish that the large wound was located primarily in the right occipital region, with involvement of the adjacent temporal and parietal lobes.

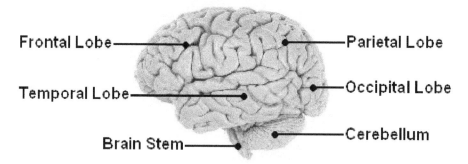

Figure 1-1: Lateral view of the human brain showing the lobes of the brain and the location of the brain stem and cerebellum (note the distinctive pattern of striation of the cerebellum).

20

The extrusion of cerebellar tissue also positions the wound at or near the bottom of the back of the President's head. As shown in Figure 1-1, the cerebellum is a distinct oval-shaped structure that sits underneath the cerebrum. Its tissue is easily identified by its unique texture, color, and striation compared to the rest of the brain. Its presence establishes that the wound was located at or near the bottom of the back of the President's skull.

THE PRESIDENT'S WOUNDS AT AUTOPSY

At Parkland Hospital the President's body was placed in a ceremonial bronze casket lined with plastic sheeting and then flown back to Washington on Air Force One. In Washington the casket was transferred to an ambulance and brought to Bethesda Naval Medical Center for an autopsy. There have been, however, persistent questions about how and when the body arrived for autopsy, the casket it was contained in, and the body's condition upon arrival.   *no practal Experiene or trade*

At Bethesda the autopsy was performed by Commander James Humes, Senior Pathologist and Director of Laboratories at Bethesda Naval Hospital, Lieutenant Colonel Pierre Finck, Chief of the Wound Ballistics Pathology Branch of the Armed Forces Institute of Pathology, and Commander J. Thorton Boswell, Chief of Pathology at Bethesda Naval Hospital. Dr. Humes acted in the capacity of chief autopsy surgeon, and signed the autopsy report, listing the cause of death as "Gunshot wound, head".

Two FBI agents were also present at the autopsy: Special Agents James Sibert and Francis O'Neill, who filed their report with the FBI shortly after the autopsy (FBI File #89-30). The report indicates that the following individuals were present at the autopsy:

- Roy Kellerman, William Greer and William O'Leary, Secret Service agents

- Admiral C.B. Holloway, Commanding Officer of the U.S. Naval Medical Center, Bethesda

- Captain James Stoner, Commanding Officer, U.S. Naval Medical School, Bethesda

- Major General Wehle, Commanding Officer of the U.S. Military District, Washington, D.C.

- Brigadier General Godfrey McHugh, Air Force Military Aide to the President

- Admiral Burkley, the President's personal physician

- Lieutenant Commander Gregg Cross

- Captain David Osborne, Chief of Surgery

- Dr. George Bakeman, U.S. Navy

- John Stringer, medical photographer

- Eight additional technicians and enlisted personnel: James Ebersole, Lloyd Raihe, J.G. Rudnicki, Paul O'Connor, J.C. Jenkins, Jerrol Crester, Edward Reed, and James Metzler

The official autopsy report is contained in Appendix A. The autopsy face sheet detailing the location of the wounds is shown in Figure 1-2. It is interesting to note that the face sheet was not included in the Autopsy Report and Supplemental Report (Commission Exhibit No. 387) that was published in the initial release of the Warren Commission Report on September 27, 1964. The autopsy face sheet appears only in the 26 volumes of testimony and exhibits that were released two months later, after Lyndon Johnson had been elected President.

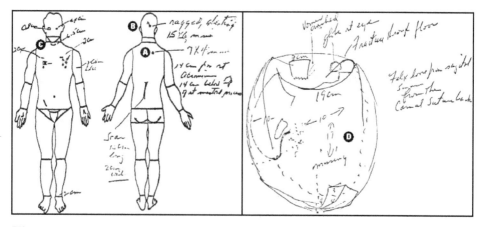

Figure 1-2. Autopsy face sheet showing the President's wounds (see text for description).

As shown in Figure 1-2, the autopsy determined that the President had sustained four wounds:

1. A small entry wound five inches down his back and just to the right of the spine (A).

2. A small entry wound at the base of the skull, just above the occipital protuberance (the small ridge at the back of the head that can be felt with a finger, typically at the level of the hairline), and an inch to the right of the midline (B).

3. A small wound at the front of the throat at the midline, just below the Adam's apple, presumed in the final autopsy report to be an exit wound (C); the nature of this wound was determined by inference during a phone call between Dr. Humes and Dr. Perry of Parkland Hospital the morning after the autopsy, when it was explained that the original wound, as noted in the Parkland doctors' reports, had been obliterated by a tracheotomy using the already open hole in the throat.

4. A large exit wound in the upper right quadrant of the head, extending across the top of the head and well into the back (D).

Each of these four wounds would eventually acquire a complex history of their own as efforts were made to characterize their perceived nature and location in support of different versions of the assassination.

The official FBI report filed by Special Agents Sibert and O'Neill stated:

"The President's body was removed from the casket *(Shipping)* in which it had been transported and was placed on the autopsy table, at which time the complete body was wrapped in a sheet and the head area contained an additional wrapping which was saturated with blood. Following the removal of the wrapping, it was ascertained that the President's clothing had been removed and it was also apparent that a tracheotomy had been performed, as well as surgery of the head area, namely, in the top of the skull. All personnel with the exception of medical officers needed in the taking of photographs and X-Rays

True

23

were requested to leave the autopsy room and remain in an adjacent room.

Upon completion of the X-Rays and photographs, the first incision was made at 8:15 p.m. X-Rays of the brain area which were developed and returned to the autopsy room disclosed a path of a missile which appeared to enter the back of the skull and the path of the disintegrated fragments could be observed along the right side of the skull. The largest section of this missile as portrayed by X-Ray appeared to be behind the right frontal sinus. The next largest fragment appeared to be at the rear of the skull at the juncture of the skull bone.

The Chief Pathologist advised approximately 40 particles of disintegrated bullet and smudges indicated that the projectile had fragmentized while passing through the skull region.

During the autopsy inspection of the area of the brain, two fragments of metal were removed by Dr. HUMES, namely, one fragment measuring 7 X 2 millimeters, which was removed from the right side of the brain. An additional fragment of metal measuring 1 X 3 millimeters was also removed from this area, both of which were placed in a glass jar containing a black metal top which were thereafter marked for identification and following the signing of a proper receipt were transported by Bureau agents to the FBI laboratory. *labeled gross material to RFR*

During the latter stages of this autopsy, Dr. HUMES located an opening which appeared to be a bullet hole which was below the shoulders and two inches to the right of the middle line of the spinal column.

This opening was probed by Dr. HUMES with the finger, at which time it was determined that the trajectory of the missile entering at this point had entered at a downward position of 45 to 60 degrees. Further probing determined that the distance traveled by this missile was a short distance inasmuch as the end of the opening could be felt with the finger.

Inasmuch as no complete bullet of any size could be located in the brain area and likewise no bullet could be located in the back or any other area of the body as determined by total body X-Rays and inspection revealing there was no point of exit, the individuals performing the autopsy were at a loss to explain why they could find no bullets. *Removed in route to Walter Reed,*

A call was made by Bureau agents to the Firearms Section of the FBI Laboratory, at which time SA CHARLES L. KILLION advised that the Laboratory had received through Secret Service Agent RICHARD JOHNSON a bullet which had reportedly been found on a stretcher in the emergency room of Parkland Hospital, Dallas, Texas. This stretcher had also contained a stethoscope and a pair of rubber gloves. Agent JOHNSON had advised the Laboratory that it had not been ascertained whether or not this was the stretcher which had been used to transport the body of President KENNEDY. Agent KILLION further described this bullet as pertaining to a 6.5 millimeter rifle which would be approximately a 25 caliber rifle and that this bullet consisted of a copper alloy full jacket.

Immediately following receipt of this information, this was made available to Dr. HUMES who advised that in his opinion this accounted for no bullet being located which had entered the back region and that since external cardiac massage had been performed at Parkland Hospital, it was entirely possible that through such movement the bullet had worked its way back out of the point of entry and had fallen on the stretcher.

Also during the latter stages of the autopsy, a piece of the skull measuring 10 X 6.5 centimeters was brought to Dr. HUMES who was instructed that this had been removed from the President's skull. Immediately this section of skull was X-Rayed, at which time it was determined by Dr. HUMES that one corner of this section revealed minute metal particles and inspection of this same area disclosed a chipping of the top portion of this piece, both of which indicated that this had been the point of exit of the bullet entering the skull region.

On the basis of the latter two developments, Dr. HUMES stated that the pattern was clear - that the one bullet had entered the President's back and had worked its way out of the body during external cardiac massage and that a second high velocity bullet had entered the rear of the skull and had fragmentized prior to exit through the top of the skull. He further pointed out that X-Rays had disclosed numerous fractures in the cranial area which he attributed to the force generated by the impact of the bullet in its passage through the brain area. He attributed the death of the President to a gunshot wound in the head.

The following is a complete listing of photographs and X-Rays taken by the medical authorities of the President's body. They were turned over to Mr. ROY KELLERMAN of the Secret Service. X-Rays were developed by the hospital, however, the photographs were delivered to Secret Service undeveloped:

> 11 X-Rays
> 22 4 X 5 color photographs
> 18 4 X 5 black and white photographs
> 1 roll of 120 film containing 5 exposures

Mr. KELLERMAN stated that these items could be made available to the FBI upon request. The portion of the skull measuring 10 X 6.5 centimeters was maintained in the custody of Dr. HUMES who stated that it also could be made available for further examination. The two metal fragments removed from the brain area were hand carried by SAs SIBERT and O'NEILL to the FBI Laboratory immediately following the autopsy and were turned over to SA KURT FRAZIER." [28]

According to Sibert and O'Neill's report, by the end of the autopsy the pathologists had concluded that one bullet had entered the President's back and lodged there, only to be dislodged by resuscitation efforts and found on a stretcher. A second shot had entered the back of the President's skull and removed the upper right quadrant of his head.

The morning after the autopsy Dr. Humes spoke with Dr. Perry of Parkland Hospital and was advised that a small bullet wound at the front of the President's throat had been obliterated by a required tracheotomy using the already open hole in the throat to try and save the President. [29]

This created a problem for the autopsy team. Oswald's rifle contained a live chambered round and only three spent cartridges were found in the sniper's nest, signifying three shots at the President. It was also known that one of the shots missed, ricocheting and hitting a bystander.

A bullet wound in the throat meant a fourth shot, which meant a second shooter, a scenario that the autopsy pathologists were apparently not allowed to consider. Dr. Humes burned his original autopsy notes (Figure 1-3) and

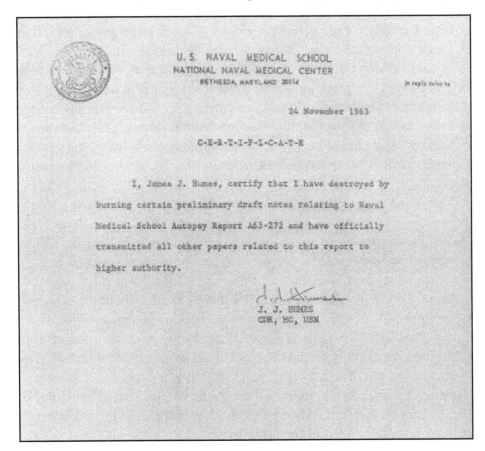

Figure 1-3. Dr. Humes certified that he burned the first draft of his autopsy notes (Commission Exhibit 397). [30]

by November 24th a new scenario had been developed: the entrance wound in the back was now found to have occurred in the President's neck, high enough to have exited the President's throat, even if shot from a height of six stories. The previously described back wound was thereafter referred to as the President's "throat wound".

In his autopsy report of November 24, 1963, Dr. Humes achieved this remarkable transmutation of a bullet wound by verbally repositioning the wound as being in two places, the first "just above the upper border of the scapula (shoulder blade)", and the second "14 cm. below the tip of the right mastoid process".

The mastoid process is located at the base of the ear, and is rarely, if ever, used as an anatomical landmark for gunshot wounds of the back.

Unfortunately for the autopsy team, Dr. Humes could not also burn the original autopsy face sheet - the original was stained with the President's blood and substitution was therefore not an option – but his verbal description would provide sufficient cover for claiming that the back wound was actually in the President's neck, no matter how ludicrous or improbable his assertion that the back wound was located 5.6 inches below the ear.

Humes' repositioned back wound was also contradicted by the physical evidence, namely the bullet holes in the clothing the President wore at the time of his death.

According to the Warren Commission Report:

"An examination of the suit jacket worn by the President by FBI Agent Frazier revealed a roughly circular hole approximately one-fourth of an inch in diameter on the rear of the coat, 5 3/8 inches below the top of the collar and 1 3/4 inches to the right of the center back seam of the coat. The hole was visible on the upper rear of the coat slightly to the right of center. Traces of copper were found in the margins of the hole and the cloth fibers around the margins were pushed inward. Those characteristics established that the hole was caused by an entering bullet. Although the precise size of the bullet could not be determined from the hole, it was consistent with having been made by a 6.5 millimeter bullet.

The shirt worn by the President contained a hole on the back side 5 3/4 inches below the top of the collar and 1 1/8 inches to the right of the middle of the back of the shirt. The hole on the rear of the shirt was approximately circular in shape and about one-fourth of an inch in diameter, with the fibers pressed inward. These factors established it as a bullet entrance hole. The relative position of the hole in the back of the suit jacket to the hole in the back of the shirt indicated that both were caused by the same penetrating missile." [31]

All of the President's clothes had been given to the Secret Service at Parkland Hospital. The autopsy pathologists had no knowledge of the location of the bullet holes in the clothing, but their original November 22nd positioning of the wound five inches down the back (as shown in Figure 1-2) was an exact match to the holes in the President's clothing.

It may also be recalled that when President Kennedy arrived at Parkland Hospital he was observed to have "obvious" damage to his right chest. [32] Such damage could not have been caused by a bullet entering the back of his neck and exiting the front, as later claimed by the autopsy team, but would be the obvious result of a gunshot wound five inches down his back, just to the right of the spine.

Further elucidation of the events at the autopsy occurred during the testimony of Dr. Finck at the 1969 New Orleans trial of Clay Shaw for conspiracy to murder the President. Appearing for the defense, Dr. Finck was questioned by Prosecutor Al Oser concerning the issue of whether the neck wound had been probed at the autopsy.

Dr. Finck: I will remind you that I was not in charge of the autopsy, that I was called -

Mr. Oser: You were a co-author of the report though, weren't you, doctor?

Dr. Finck: Wait. I was called as a consultant to look at these wounds; that doesn't mean I am running the show.

Mr. Oser: Was Dr. Humes running the show?

Dr. Finck: Well I heard Dr. Humes stating that – he said, "Who's in charge here?" and I heard an Army general, I don't remember his name, stating, "I am." You must understand that in those circumstances, there were law enforcement officers, military people with various ranks and you have to coordinate the operation according to directions.

FINCK?

Mr. Oser: But you were one of the three qualified pathologists standing at the autopsy table, were you not, doctor?

Dr. Finck: Yes, I was.

Mr. Oser: Was this Army general a qualified pathologist?

Dr. Finck: No.

Mr. Oser: Was he a doctor?

Dr. Finck: No, not to my knowledge.

Mr. Oser: Can you give me his name, colonel?

Dr. Finck: No, I can't. I don't remember.

Mr. Oser: Do you happen to have the photographs and X-rays taken of President Kennedy's body at the time of the autopsy and shortly thereafter? Do you?

Dr. Finck: I do not have X-rays or photographs of President Kennedy with me.

Mr. Oser: How many other military personnel were present at the autopsy room?

Dr. Finck: That autopsy room was quite crowded. It is a small autopsy room, and when you are called in circumstances like that to look at the wound of the President of the United States who is dead, you don't look around too much to ask people for their names and take notes on who they are and how many there are. I did not do so. The room was crowded with military and civilian personnel and federal agents, Secret Service agents, FBI agents, for part of the autopsy, but I cannot give you a precise breakdown as regards the attendance of the people in that autopsy room at Bethesda Naval Hospital.

Mr. Oser: Colonel, did you feel that you had to take orders from this Army general that was there directing the autopsy?

Dr. Finck: No, because there were others, there were admirals.

Mr. Oser: There were admirals?

Dr. Finck: Oh, yes, there were admirals, and when you are a lieutenant colonel in the Army you just follow orders, and at the end of the autopsy we were specifically told – as I recall it, it was by Admiral Kinney, the surgeon of the Navy – this is subject to verification – we were specifically told not to discuss the case.

Mr. Oser: Did you have occasion to dissect the track of that particular bullet in the victim as it lay on the autopsy table?

Dr. Finck: I did not dissect the track in the neck.

Mr. Oser: Why?

Dr. Finck: This leads us into the disclosure of medical records.

Mr. Oser: Your Honor, I would like an answer from the colonel and I would ask the Court to so direct.

The Court: That is correct, you should answer, doctor.

Dr. Finck: We didn't remove the organs of the neck.

Mr. Oser: Why not, doctor?

Dr. Finck: For the reason that we were told to examine the head wounds and the -

Mr. Oser: Are you saying that someone told you not to dissect the track?

The Court: Let him finish his answer.

Dr. Finck: I was told that the family wanted an examination of the head, as I recall, the head and chest, but prosecutors in this autopsy didn't remove the organs of the neck, to my recollection.

Mr. Oser: You have said they did not. I want to know why didn't you as an autopsy pathologist attempt to ascertain the track through the body which you had on the autopsy table in trying to ascertain the cause or causes of death? Why?

Dr. Finck: I had the cause of death.

Mr. Oser: Why did you not trace the track of the wound?

Dr. Finck: As I recall I didn't remove these organs from the neck.

Mr. Oser: I didn't hear you.

Dr. Finck: I examined the wounds but I didn't remove the organs of the neck.

Mr. Oser: You said you didn't do this. I am asking you why you didn't do this as a pathologist?

Dr. Finck: From what I recall I looked at the trachea, there was a tracheotomy wound the best I can remember, but I didn't dissect or remove these organs.

Mr. Oser: Your Honor, I would ask Your Honor to direct the witness to answer my question. I will ask you the question one more time:

Why did you not dissect the track of the bullet wound that you have described today and you saw at the time of the autopsy at the time you examined the body? Why? I ask you to answer the question.

Dr. Finck: As I recall I was told not to, but I don't remember by whom. [33]

THE PRESIDENT'S WOUNDS
IN THE WARREN COMMISSION REPORT

The Warren Commission Report contains several exhibits showing the Commission's version of how the President was shot. Figure 1-4 shows the Commission's depiction of the President's alleged entry wounds compared to their original autopsy locations as recorded the evening of November 22, 1963.

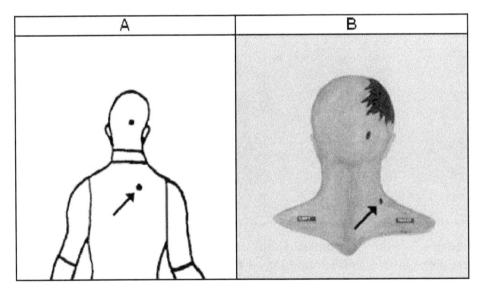

Figure 1-4. Location of the President's entrance wounds as determined at autopsy the evening of November 22, 1963 (A), and Commission Exhibit 386, the Commission's version of the President's wounds showing the repositioning of the back wound into the neck (B). The original location shown on the left is consistent with the bullet holes in the President's clothing.

In its report the Commission makes frequent reference to an amateur home movie of the assassination made by Abraham Zapruder (known as the Zapruder film). This establishes that the Commission had access to the film, and had viewed it. The Commission asserted that one of the sixth floor sniper's bullets entered the base of the President's skull and then exploded out of the top of his head in Frame 313 of the Zapruder film (in what came to be known as the "head shot"), creating a scenario that required the President to be facing the floor of his limousine at the time of the shot.

Figure 1-5 shows the Warren Commission version of the "head shot", compared to the preceding frame of the Zapruder film (312), as well as the path of the bullet from the sixth floor sniper's nest. The figure clearly demonstrates that the shot could not have occurred in the manner claimed by the Commission. President Kennedy was not facing the floor of the limousine as shown in Commission Exhibit 388, and the shot descended at too steep an angle to have exited out of the top of his head.

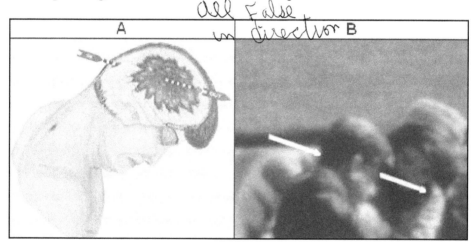

Figure 1-5. Warren Commission Exhibit 388 (A) showing the Commission's version of how a shot to the base of the President's skull exploded out of the top of his head, and (B) the President's actual position in Zapruder Frame 312, immediately before the "head shot" in Frame 313. Note that in the Commission's version the President was facing the limousine floor, when in fact he was almost upright. Zapruder Frame 312 shows that a bullet entering the base of the President's skull would have passed underneath the President's brain and exited at the level of the eyes.

34

The Commission was undaunted by the lack of correspondence between their public assertions and the forensic evidence. In an attempt to prove the Commission's lone-sniper-three-shots theory and reconcile their version of the wounds, Assistant Counsel Arlen Specter proposed the single bullet theory, wherein the undamaged bullet found on the stretcher in Dallas (Figure 1-6) had struck the President in the back on a downward path, reversed direction upward to exit the President's throat, and then continued on to cause the multiple wounds observed in Governor Connally. [34]

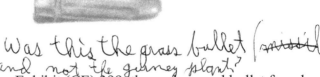

Was this the grass bullet (pristine) and not the gurney plant?

Figure 1-6. Commission Exhibit (CE) 399, the undamaged bullet found on a stretcher at Parkland Hospital.

Many found this path to be highly improbable, if not impossible, and thus the single bullet theory was dubbed the "magic" bullet theory by its detractors. It eventually proved to be the "impossible" bullet theory, because the mass of the undamaged bullet found on the stretcher plus the mass of the bullet fragments found in Governor Connally's wrist exceeded the mass of a whole bullet. The bullet was pristine and could not possibly have left all of the fragments found in Governor Connally's body.

Counselor Specter should have known better than to advance such a theory because he himself had questioned Dr. Finck on this point during Finck's testimony before the Commission:

Mr. Specter: And could it have been the bullet (CE 399) which inflicted the wound on Governor Connally's right wrist?

Dr. Finck: No; for the reason that there are too many fragments described in that wrist. [35]

In his testimony before the Commission Dr. Humes also told Specter that CE 399 could not have inflicted the observed wounds:

Commander Humes: …The reason I believe it most unlikely that this missile (CE 399) could have inflicted either of these wounds (President Kennedy's head wound or Governor Connally's wrist wound) is that this missile is basically intact; its jacket appears to me to be intact, and I do not understand how it could possibly have left fragments in either of these locations. [36]

CHAPTER 2

THE OFFICIAL VERSIONS II: THE CLARK PANEL

Deep State Power Lawyer

Popular discontent with the Warren Commission Report had been growing since its release, and in 1968 the Attorney General of the United States, Ramsey Clark, appointed a panel of four doctors to examine the photographs and X-rays taken at the autopsy and render an opinion as to the cause and manner of the President's death. This came to be known as the Clark Panel.

Clark asked the President of the College of American Pathologists and three university presidents to recommend the pathologists who would constitute the Panel. The Panel was comprised of:

1. Dr. Russell S. Fisher, Professor of Forensic Pathology, University of Maryland, and Chief Medical Examiner of the State of Maryland, nominated by Dr. Oscar B. Hunter, President of the College of American Pathologists.

2. Dr. William H. Carnes, Professor of Pathology, University of Utah, Member of the Medical Examiners Commission for the State of Utah, nominated by Dr. J.E. Wallace Sterling, President of Stanford University.

3. Dr. Russell H. Morgan, Professor of Radiology, School of Medicine, and Professor of Radiological Science, School of Hygiene and Public Health, Johns Hopkins University, nominated by Dr. Lincoln Gordon, President of Johns Hopkins University.

4. Dr. Alan R. Moritz, Professor of Pathology, Case Western Reserve University, and former Professor of Forensic Medicine,

Harvard University, nominated by Dr. John A. Hannah, President of Michigan State University.

Clark asked Mr. Bruce Bromley, a member of the New York Bar who had been nominated by the President of the American Bar Association, to serve as legal counsel to the Panel and assist in the preparation of the final report.

The Panel's final report solemnly declares that "no one of the undersigned has had any previous connection with prior investigations of, or reports on this matter, and each has acted with complete and unbiased independence free of preconceived views as to the correctness of the medical conclusions reached in the 1963 Autopsy Report and Supplementary Report." *

The Panel was asked to examine the Kennedy assassination photographs, X-ray films, and other documents stored in the National Archives, and evaluate their significance relative to the medical conclusions contained in the assassination autopsy report. They met February 26 – 27, 1968, and the report was completed and signed by the following April.

The Panel noted that the autopsy report stated that X-rays had been made of the entire body, but an inventory of the X-rays in the Archives disclosed that X-rays of the lower arms, wrists, hands, and lower legs, ankles and feet were missing.

The Panel agreed with the Warren Commission that the President had been struck twice from behind. Using language virtually identical to the autopsy report, they found that one of these shots struck the President in the back of the neck, exiting from the front. In agreement with the Warren Commission, the Panel stated that the neck wound was situated 14 cm. (5.6 inches) below the right mastoid process, located at the base of the right ear.

However, unlike the autopsy pathologists, the Panel had access to the

---

* Bruce Bromley was an employee of former CIA Director and Warren Commissioner Allen Dulles' law firm, Sullivan and Cromwell. There have been allegations that all three university presidents used in the creation of the Panel had direct ties to the CIA, and that Dr. Russell Fisher later falsified the cause of death of high level CIA counterintelligence operative John Paisley, ruling that the right handed Paisley committed suicide by shooting himself in the head behind his left ear. Paisley had been tied to the infamous Watergate break-in. [1-3]

dress shirt that the President was wearing at the time of the assassination. They determined that the bullet hole in the shirt was 14 cm. below the top of the shirt's collar.

The Panel was thus confronted with the logical impossibility that the President's shirt collar and right mastoid process were both 14 cm. above the wound, indicating that they were both in approximately the same place. Typically the distance between the mastoid process and the top of a buttoned shirt collar is three to four vertical inches.

The only conclusion that can be drawn is that either the bullet hole measurement of the shirt was incorrect, which is unlikely, or that the measurement of the distance between the wound and the mastoid process was incorrect. In any event it is not possible that the shirt collar and the mastoid process were both 14 cm. above the President's back wound.

In 1963 the autopsy pathologists determined that the President had an entrance wound at the base of his skull, "just above the occipital protuberance".

In contrast to the original autopsy report, the Clark Panel maintained that the entrance wound in the President's head was not at the base of his skull, but was actually located 100 mm. (4 inches) higher, near the top of the skull. According to the Panel, the back of the President's head was otherwise undamaged, with most of the damage to the skull contained in the right frontal and parietal areas. [4]

Despite their mandate to examine all relevant documentation, including the Warren Commission Report, the Panel did not comment on the conspicuous differences between their findings and those of the autopsy pathologists and the Warren Commission.

As shown in the Warren Commission Report, all of the Parkland doctors who saw the President's wounds described a huge gaping hole in the back of his head. The autopsy pathologists similarly described a huge hole extending well into the back of the President's head. Warren Commission Exhibit 386 shows a large wound extending well into the back of the President's head (Figure 1-4B).

In contrast, the Clark Panel found that there was no damage to the back of the President's head, and made no comment on the discrepancy.

The autopsy pathologists and the Warren Commission determined that the President had an entrance wound at the base of his skull. The Clark Panel found that the entrance wound was four inches higher, at the top of his head, and made no comment on the discrepancy.

Many believe that the Clark Panel was created in response to New Orleans District Attorney Jim Garrison's emerging investigation into the activities of Lee Harvey Oswald in New Orleans during the summer preceding the assassination. Garrison had been attempting to secure access to the autopsy documentation that had been deposited in the National Archives. Although the report of the Clark Panel was completed by April 1968, it was not released until January 16, 1969, the day before James B. Rhodes, archivist of the United States, was to appear in court to show cause as to why he should not turn over the requested materials to Garrison. [5]

CHAPTER 3

THE OFFICIAL VERSIONS III: THE HOUSE SELECT COMMITTEE ON ASSASSINATIONS

In 1975 the American public had the opportunity to view the Zapruder film for the first time on Geraldo Rivera's television variety show. Millions watched in horror and revulsion as the film showed the President's head rocketed back and to the left by a bullet that shattered the upper right quadrant of his skull. The resulting outcry and general disbelief in the findings of the Warren Commission led the United States House of Representatives to adopt a resolution creating the House Select Committee on Assassinations in 1976. Its designated purpose was to examine the assassination of President Kennedy and that of the Reverend Martin Luther King in 1968. The Committee was created four months before the end of the congressional session, when it would then expire and have to be renewed by the next Congress in order to complete its work.

The Committee got off to an inauspicious start when Congressman Henry Gonzalez became the Committee Chairman and engaged in fratricidal bureaucratic warfare with Chief Counsel Richard Sprague. Eventually both were forced to resign. Gonzalez was replaced by Congressman Louis Stokes, and Sprague was replaced by Robert Blakey, a professor at Cornell University who had specialized in organized crime while employed by the Department of Justice. [1]

The Committee's investigation of the Kennedy assassination focused on
ʿs:

1. Identity of the assassin(s).

2. Existence of a foreign or domestic conspiracy to assassinate the President.

3. Performance of federal and local law enforcement before, during and after the assassination.

4. Adequacy of the methods, results and conclusions of the Warren Commission.

In his remarks prior to the testimony of medical illustrator Ida Dox, Chief Counsel Blakey gave a summary of the medical issues before the Committee:

"The handling of President Kennedy's treatment and autopsy – first in Texas and then in Washington – by the doctors, the Warren Commission, and by the President's family, has given rise to more questions touching on his assassination than any other single aspect of the investigation. The facts of what happened and the questions that have arisen out of those facts merit the closest attention.

The first doctors to attend the President at Parkland Hospital were Malcolm Perry and Charles J. Carrico. According to each, they observed a massive head wound and a small, circular wound in the neck just below the Adam's apple. Later, they referred to it as an 'entry wound.' Dr. Perry performed a tracheotomy to help the President breathe. The incision was made at the throat wound, making it subsequently difficult to determine the nature of the wound or even to notice its existence.

Other Parkland doctors have differed dramatically in their descriptions of the head wound.* Dr. Robert McClelland, in a

---

* The Parkland doctors did not differ dramatically in their descriptions of the head wound. In clinical reports filed within hours of the assassination they uniformly described the President as having a large gaping hole in the back of his head. Dr. Perry stated that "a large wound of the right posterior cranium was noted, exposing severely lacerated brain". Dr. Carrico wrote

written report dated November 22, 1963, described it as 'a massive head and brain injury from a gunshot wound of the left temple.' Dr. William Kemp Clark said he observed a large gaping hole in the rear of the President's head.

The Parkland doctors worked on the President for about 20 minutes. They did not examine his back, so they could not have been aware of a wound there. The only head wound they say they saw was the massive one they described. Their job, of course, was to administer emergency treatment, not to measure the location of wounds or to determine that all wounds had been accounted for. The Parkland doctors' duties extended only up until the time of the death of the President.

Efforts to save the President were futile; Dr. Clark pronounced him dead at 1 p.m., central standard time. It was a formality. The President was beyond help before he arrived at the hospital.

The doctors who examined Governor Connally were Robert Shaw, Charles Gregory, and George Shires. They described the wounds to his back, chest, wrist, and thigh. The Governor, at first listed as critical, fully recovered.

---

that there was an "attempt to control slow oozing from cerebral and cerebellar tissue". In testimony before the Warren Commission Dr. McClelland stated that "the right posterior portion of the skull had been extremely blasted. It had been shattered, apparently, by the force of the shot so that the parietal bone was protruding up through the scalp and seemed to be fractured almost along its right posterior half, as well as some of the occipital bone being fractured in its lateral half, and this sprung open the bones that I mentioned in such a way that you could actually look down into the skull cavity itself and see that probably a third or so, at least, of the brain tissue, posterior cerebral tissue and some of the cerebellar tissue had been blasted out". [2] The Parkland doctors reiterated that President Kennedy had a large hole in the back of his head in a 2013 book entitled *We Were There: Revelations from the Dallas Doctors Who Attended to JFK on November 22, 1963*.

After the President was declared dead, his body was taken to Air Force One for the flight back to Washington. On the return flight, Mrs. Kennedy decided to have the autopsy performed at Bethesda Naval Hospital, since the President had served in the Navy. Comdr. James J. Humes was appointed chief autopsy surgeon. He, in turn, chose Drs. J. Thorton Boswell and Pierre A. Finck to assist him. The autopsy began at 8 p.m. eastern standard time. Other doctors, laboratory technicians, Secret Service and FBI agents and military personnel were in attendance. Members of the Kennedy family and friends remained in the tower suite of the hospital.

Preliminary X-rays failed to detect the presence of a missile in the President's body. Commander Humes was then given authority to conduct a full autopsy by Adm. Calvin B. Galloway and Dr. George Burkley, the White House physician.

Dr. Humes first determined that a missile had entered the rear of the head and exited at the top right side of the skull, resulting in a large exit wound and leaving tiny metallic particles throughout the brain.

Next, he found a wound he determined had entered the upper back. Pathologists tried to probe this wound, but they could only detect a pathway that extended a few inches. They could not find a point of exit. Despite the uncertainty over the missile track, Dr. Humes decided not to dissect the track through the neck.

At about this time, Dr. Humes was informed by FBI agents that a bullet had been discovered on a stretcher in the emergency room at Parkland. He and the other pathologists tentatively decided the bullet had penetrated a few inches into the President's back and had been dislodged during emergency treatment at the hospital.

During the autopsy, pieces of bone discovered in the Presidential limousine were brought to Bethesda, where they were determined to have been part of the President's skull.

Dr. Humes made note of the tracheotomy incision. The pathologists examined most major organs of the President's body. X-rays and photographs were taken. The brain was retained for future examination; slides were extracted from tissue organs and sections. The autopsy ended at about 11 p.m. eastern standard time.

On the morning of Saturday, November 23, Dr. Humes spoke by telephone with Dr. Perry in Dallas, who explained that he had made the tracheotomy incision through a small, circular throat wound. Dr. Humes then theorized it was an exit corresponding to the entry wound in the upper back, and he reflected this belief in his autopsy report filed November 24.

All participants in the autopsy were under naval orders – not lifted until the select committee began its investigation – to be silent as to its results, but rumors began to fly anyway, and confusing news accounts soon began to appear. The effect of these erroneous news accounts on public perceptions is important to emphasize. Here is a sampling from the New York Times:

November 23: The President suffered an entrance wound in the Adam's apple and a massive head wound in the head.

December 17: The FBI had concluded one bullet had struck the President in the right temple and another had hit where the right shoulder joins the neck.

December 19: The pathologists had determined a bullet had lodged in the back, a second had struck the right rear of the head.

J. Edgar Hoover, the Director of the FBI, submitted the Bureau's report of the assassination to the Warren Commission on December 9, and a supplement to it was filed on January 13, 1964. They reflected the preliminary observations of the FBI agents, who had attended the autopsy.

By early February, the theory that one bullet had traversed President Kennedy's back and throat wounds and caused Governor Connally's wounds – the so called single bullet theory – began to emerge. At this time, and for several months to come, members of the Warren Commission and its staff were taking testimony from the doctors who had attended the President and who had participated in the autopsy. The Warren Commission and its staff had also viewed the Zapruder film. As far as is known, however, no member of the Commission, or its staff, ever carefully examined the autopsy X-rays or photos, although Chief Justice Warren is reported to have seen them.

In September 1964, the Warren Commission issued its report, in which it concluded the President had been struck by two bullets, one in the back and one in the rear of the skull, as the autopsy report had indicated. Although it used carefully guarded language, the Commission concluded that the bullet that exited the President's throat also caused all of Governor Connally's wounds.

Finally, the Commission said the bullet that was found on the stretcher at Parkland Hospital was the one that hit both the President and Governor Connally. This bullet, known by its exhibit number, CE 399, has come to be known as the pristine bullet.

Not long after publication of the Warren report, criticisms of its findings began to appear. In 1966, Edward Jay Epstein, in Inquest, revealed that the FBI report of December 9, 1963, stated that the missile that entered the President's back did not exit – this, in spite of the fact that the FBI had access to Dr. Humes' written report indicating otherwise.

In addition, in 1966, Mark Lane published his 'Rush to Judgement.' He quoted the early comments of several doctors at Parkland, in which they described the throat wound 'as one of entry.' Lane then argued that if the President was hit both from the front and back, there had to be more than one assassin. Lane also criticized the 'single bullet' theory, suggesting that it had been devised by the Warren Commission to explain how one assassin could have inflicted all the wounds in the requisite time period. As the 'single bullet' theory fell, so, argued Lane, the specter of two gunmen rose.

In 1967, Josiah Thompson, in 'Six Seconds in Dallas,' proposed that the President had been struck simultaneously by two shots, one from the rear and one from the front.

In October 1966, the autopsy materials, which had been, up until that time, retained by the Kennedy family, were transferred to the custody of the National Archives under a restrictive deed of gift that sharply limited public access to them. In November 1966, the autopsy pathologists were asked by the Department of Justice to review the X-rays and photographs. This was the first time they had ever reviewed the photographs. Nevertheless, they concluded they were consistent with their original autopsy findings.

In 1968, Acting Attorney General Ramsey Clark convened a panel of medical experts for the purpose of making an independent review of the X-rays and photos. The panel confirmed the autopsy findings as to the number of wounds and the general direction from which the shots came, but it differed with the pathologists at Bethesda on one important point: it said that the wound in the rear of the President's head was 10 centimeters above where it had been placed by the autopsy.

In 1975, the Rockefeller Commission asked still another panel of experts to review the photographic evidence. The findings concurred with those of the panel appointed by Clark.

In 1976, the select committee was, of course, charged by the House of Representatives to undertake its investigation into the assassination of President Kennedy. The committee recognized that it, too, was obligated to examine all of the medical issues that had arisen over the years.

They include: (1) The number of bullets that struck President Kennedy and Governor Connally; (2) the number of wounds each man received, their locations and whether they were wounds of entry or exit; (3) the 10-centimeter discrepancy in the location of the

47

wound to the rear of the President's head; (4) the course of the so-called pristine bullet through both President Kennedy and Governor Connally; (5) the apparent backward motion of the President's head, as shown in the Zapruder film, as he is hit by the fatal bullet; (6) the possibility that the President was struck in both the rear and the front of the head; (7) the statements of the Parkland doctors concerning President Kennedy's wounds; (8) the authenticity of the autopsy X-rays and photographs; (9) the competence and the validity of the autopsy, including an allegation that the pathologists were ordered to perform an incomplete examination.

The committee has convened a panel of forensic pathologists to evaluate and interpret the medical evidence. It consists of two groups of doctors – one that had previously reviewed the autopsy photographs and X-rays and one that had not.

Panel members who had previously reviewed the evidence are:

Dr. Werner Spitz, medical examiner of Detroit, Mich.

Dr. Cyril H. Wecht, coroner of Allegheny County, Pa.

Dr. James T. Weston, chief medical investigator, University of New Mexico School of Medicine, Albuquerque, N. Mex.

Panel members who had not previously reviewed the evidence are:

Dr. John I. Coe, chief medical examiner of Hennepin County, Minn.

Dr. Joseph H. Davis, chief medical examiner of Dade County, Fla.

Dr. Joseph S. Loquvam, director of the Institute of Forensic Sciences, Oakland, Calif.

Dr. Charles S. Petty, chief medical examiner, Dallas County, Tex.

Dr. Earl Rose, professor of pathology, University of Iowa, Iowa City, Iowa.

The moderator of the panel is Dr. Michael M. Baden, chief medical examiner of New York City.

The panel was asked by the committee to undertake four fundamental assignments:

One, to determine whether there are basic conclusions in the field of forensic pathology on which most, or all, of the panel members could agree.

Two, to perform a detailed critique of the autopsy of President Kennedy.

Three, to write a report of its findings.

Four, to make recommendations for pursuing matters outside the expertise of forensic pathologists.

The committee has arranged to have the two groups of medical experts express their views in a single report with the stipulation that, should any member hold a dissenting opinion, it would be stated in the body of the report.

The committee has also conducted a comprehensive investigation in an attempt to locate missing materials, that is, materials missing from the National Archives, including a steel container alleged to have contained the President's brain which was removed during the autopsy.

All persons, either directly or indirectly, involved in the chain of custody of the autopsy materials have been either interviewed or deposed. The total number of persons interviewed or deposed exceeds 30. The committee has also contacted the Kennedy family.

Despite these efforts, the committee has not been able to determine what precisely happened to the missing materials. A family spokesman, however, did indicate that Attorney General Robert F. Kennedy expressed concern that these materials could conceivably be placed on public display many years from then and that he wished to prevent it.

The spokesman indicated that in his judgment, the materials were destroyed and cannot be recovered. The committee has determined that the materials were not buried with the body of the President at reinterment. The committee has not obtained any other relevant information on this issue." [3]

The Committee then took testimony from medical illustrator Ida Dox, who testified that she was assigned to create exact copies of four of the autopsy pictures in the National Archives, as well as other illustrations for the Committee. The four illustrations were used in lieu of the actual autopsy photographs themselves. The Committee declared that the purpose of this strategy was to avoid invading the privacy of the Kennedy family that might occur with the release of the actual autopsy photographs, but it is clear that the use of medical illustrations instead of photographs could obscure modifications that had been made to the photographs in their production.

After taking testimony from dental identification expert Dr. Lowell Levine and photography expert Calvin McCamy, the Committee heard from Dr. Michael Baden. In his testimony Dr. Baden stated on behalf of the panel of forensic pathologists that:

1. The panel had reviewed a wide variety of materials that were supplied to them, including a full set of autopsy documentation, Dr. Finck's reports and testimony at the New Orleans trial of Clay Shaw, the Warren Commission testimony of the Parkland Hospital doctors and autopsy pathologists, Committee staff interviews, ballistics materials, Secret Service and FBI reports, and motion pictures and still photographs from the assassination.

2. The essential conclusions of the panel were unanimously agreed to by eight of the nine members of the panel, with Dr. Cyril Wecht expressing dissent on some important aspects of the conclusions.

3. President Kennedy was hit by two bullets, one of which entered his upper right back, and the other which entered high on the back of his head (Figures 3-1 and 3-2).

4. In the President's jacket and shirt there are perforations that correspond to the location of an entrance wound in the President's

upper right back.

5. X-rays of the President's neck and upper chest are consistent with a bullet passing through the body and no longer being present.

6. The Warren Commission placed the entry of the President's back wound two inches too high.

7. Autopsy photographs of the back of the President's head show an entrance wound at the top of the head, near the cowlick, and a fragment of extraneous dried brain tissue near the hairline of the President; the corresponding exit wound occurred at the upper right front on the President's skull (Figure 3-1).

8. The medical panel unanimously concluded that the entrance wound on the President's head was four inches above the point indicated on the official autopsy report.

9. The medical panel unanimously concluded that Governor Connally had: i) an entrance wound of the right lateral back with a corresponding exit wound in his chest, ii) an entrance wound of the right wrist with a corresponding exit from the front surface of the wrist, and iii) an entrance wound in his thigh with a subsequent dislodgment of the bullet; all three wounds were caused by the same bullet.

10. The bullet that caused all of the injuries to Governor Connally is the same bullet that struck President Kennedy in the back and exited out of the front of his neck, namely Warren Commission Exhibit 399.

11. The medical panel noted several deficiencies with respect to the manner in which the President's autopsy was performed, including: i) improper assumption of jurisdiction of the body, ii) deficiencies in the qualifications of the autopsy pathologists, iii) failure of the autopsy pathologists to contact the Parkland doctors in a timely manner, iv) failure to examine the President's clothing, v) failure to properly document the President's injuries, vi) failure to properly preserve evidence, and vii) failure to conduct a complete autopsy.

12. No bullet struck the President from the front or the side.

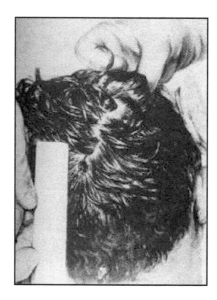

Figure 3-1. House Select Committee on Assassinations Exhibit F-48, a medical drawing of an autopsy photograph in the National Archives showing the back of the President's head. The 1978 forensic pathology panel claimed that the 1963 autopsy missed the bullet hole shown near the middle of the photograph. The panel further suggested that the autopsy pathologists mistakenly thought that the dried brain fragment at the bottom of the photograph was a bullet hole, despite the fact that the autopsy pathologists had access to developed X-rays at the autopsy. Note that except for the alleged bullet hole, the back of the President's head is otherwise undisturbed, despite the observations by Parkland Hospital doctors, Secret Service staff, the autopsy pathologists, and the Warren Commission that the President had a huge gaping hole in the back of his head.

Dr. Baden was asked about the discrepancy between the 1963 autopsy pathologists' location of the entrance of the President's head wound at the base of his skull, and the 1978 forensic pathology panel's conclusion that the entrance wound was actually four inches higher, at the top of the skull. Dr. Baden stated that the finding was based solely on the photographs and X-rays that were provided to the panel (Figure 3-3), and he noted that the autopsy pathologists had placed the wound at approximately the same location as a piece of dried brain tissue on the photographs, suggesting that the autopsy pathologists had been fooled, along with the autopsy technical

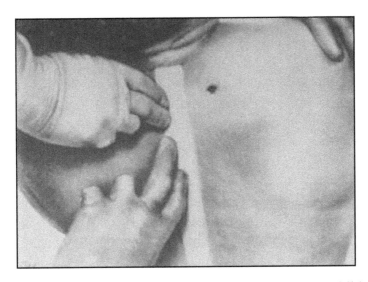

Figure 3-2. House Select Committee on Assassinations Exhibit F-20, a medical drawing of an autopsy photograph in the National Archives showing the wound in the President's back. The positioning of the President's body at the time the photograph was taken is unknown, but it is clear that a bullet entering the President's back at this location from a shot fired from the sixth floor of the Texas School Book Depository could not have exited the President's throat. Author Harrison Livingstone studied this and similar photographs in the National Archives and observed that another photograph of the back wound that included the head region did not show the bullet wound displayed in Figure 3-1.

staff, physicians, and military commanders present, into mistaking a piece of dried brain tissue for a bullet hole.[4] Baden noted that the medical panel's observations were in agreement with those of the Clark Panel and the Rockefeller Commission, who had drawn the same conclusions after viewing the same photographs and X-rays.

Dr. Baden was then asked about the Warren Commission testimony of Dr. Shaw, one of the Parkland Hospital doctors who had treated Governor Connally. Dr. Shaw had objected to the single bullet theory before the Commission. Dr. Baden said that Dr. Shaw's objection was based on the recollections of Governor Connally and Mrs. Connally. Governor Connally had testified before the Commission that he had heard the first shot and was

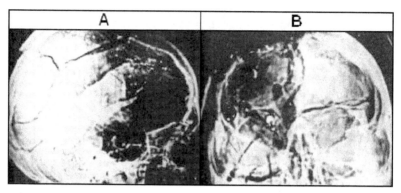

Figure 3-3. House Select Committee on Assassinations Exhibits F-53 (A) and F-56 (B), autopsy X-rays in the National Archives showing the right front of the President's skull to be completely obliterated. Figure 3-4 below shows an autopsy photograph in the National Archives that demonstrates that the President's face was left completely intact, whereas the X-rays above show the right upper portion of his face to be completely destroyed. The X-rays were cropped in a manner that precludes dental identification.

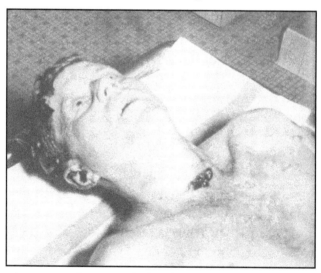

Figure 3-4. Autopsy photograph in the National Archives showing the President's face to be completely intact, whereas the X-rays in Figure 3-3 show a significant portion to be completely destroyed. A medical drawing of this photograph was created and used in the Committee's report (HSCA Exhibit F-36), but was cropped to remove the President's face, with only the neck and upper chest appearing.

turning to see the President when he was struck. Mrs. Connally had testified that she heard the first shot, had turned to see the President clutching at his throat, and after that had observed Governor Connally being struck. Dr. Baden found that Dr. Shaw's reasoning was not valid because it was based on eyewitness accounts instead of scientific evidence. [5]

When questioned about the rapid movement of the President's head back and to the left after being shot, Dr. Baden stated that predicting how a head would react in response to being shot is beyond the capabilities of medical science. Questioned about the single bullet theory in light of the bullet fragments extracted from Governor Connally, as well as those still remaining in Connally's wrist, Dr. Baden replied that the observed fragments could have come from CE 399.

CE 399 showed no evidence of fragmentation. Dr. Baden was also questioned about the fact that in the Zapruder film Governor Connally can be seen holding his hat in his right hand well after President Kennedy has been hit, indicating that Kennedy and Connally were struck by separate bullets. Dr. Baden suggested that Governor Connally was holding his hat because he did not know his wrist was injured, and that it was the opinion of the forensic pathology panel that the same bullet went through President Kennedy and Governor Connally, in part, because there was no evidence of another bullet.

The Committee took dissenting testimony from Dr. Cyril Wecht, who expressed disagreement with the single bullet theory, and therefore, in his opinion, with the idea that there was only one shooter. Dr. Wecht expressed dismay with the lack of interest in performing controlled experiments to determine if a single bullet could have caused all of the described injuries and emerged in the same condition as CE 399, i.e. undeformed and in nearly pristine condition. He also noted Governor Connally's testimony and belief that he was struck by a shot other than the first shot to hit the President, and he reviewed Warren Commission exhibits showing the degree of bullet deformation that occurs after a bullet strikes a rib. Dr. Wecht found the idea that CE 399 was consistent with the wounds to President Kennedy and Governor Connally to be "absolutely false". [6]

The interest of the forensic pathology panel in promoting the single bullet theory presented a number of obvious problems that the panel had to mitigate or ignore, namely i) the fact that in the Zapruder film Governor

Connally displayed no signs of injury until well after the President had been shot in the back, ii) the improbable course of the bullet as it continued on to hit Governor Connally, iii) the lack of deformation of the bullet as it struck several bones in Governor Connally, and iv) the numerous fragments that were deposited in Governor Connally, despite the lack of fragmentation of the bullet.

In addition to these factors, the forensic pathology panel positioned the President's back wound two inches lower than the Warren Commission, making it more difficult to sustain a scenario that has the bullet emerging from the front of the President's neck, just below the Adam's apple. To this end, the panel posited that the President was leaning forward when he was struck, thus lowering the front of his neck relative to the back. This point was addressed in the testimony of panel member Dr. Charles Petty before the Committee. Dr. Petty stated that he believed that President Kennedy and Governor Connally were struck by the same bullet, and that:

"I think it is necessary at this point to sum up, in a sense, the flight of the bullet and its effect on those it struck. The bullet that struck the late President in the upper right back area and then went on to penetrate the soft structures of the neck and to exit in the front of the neck was, as has been indicated already, traveling in a somewhat upward direction anatomically speaking.

Anatomists many years ago decided – the better to understand each other – to place a body in a specific position and to relate all of the descriptions of the landmarks of the body to the body in that position. That position actually is a person standing erect facing forward with both palms turned forward. This is the anatomic position and in tracing the in-shoot wound on the back of the late President and connecting it with a more-or-less straight line with the out-shoot wound on the front of the neck, the bullet will have followed a slightly upward direction. But the President was not upright at the time he was shot, he was certainly not in the anatomic position, and this explains, I believe, the objection that Dr. Wecht had and his argument that he could not understand how the bullet pursued a downward track from where it was discharged, then an upward track in the President and then a downward track into Mr. Connally." [7]

Dr. Petty apparently did not consult the Zapruder film before formulating his rationale to support the single bullet theory. The Zapruder film shows that the President was upright when he was struck in the back (Figure 3-5).

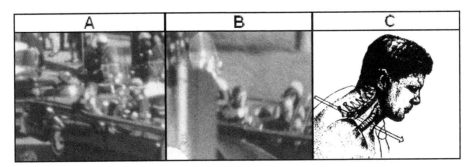

Figure 3-5. Zapruder Frames 188 (A) and 226 (B), during which the President is shot in the back. His hands are beginning to rise toward his throat in Zapruder Frame 226, indicating that he has already been shot. At no point from Frame 188 through Frame 226 (approximately two seconds) was the President observed being tilted forward. Panel C shows the House Select Committee version of events, which had the President tilted forward at a 45 degree angle when hc was shot in the back; the forward tilt was required for the bullet to enter the President's back and exit the front of his throat.

The Committee went on to take testimony from witnesses and experts in various fields, including ballistics, science and technology, photographic and handwriting analysis, the FBI, the Secret Service, the CIA, foreign intelligence, Cuban affairs, the Warren Commission, and Jack Ruby's substantial ties to organized crime.

The Committee also heard testimony from acoustics experts, who were introduced by Chief Counsel Blakey:

"In September 1977 the committee learned of the existence of a Dallas police tape, one that had recorded the sounds of the assassination from the transmitter of a motorcycle policeman who had accidentally left his microphone switch in the on position.

There was immediate hope that by scientifically enhancing the tape, the sound of the shots could be made audible.

The committee was told by the Dallas Police Department that it thought that all of its assassination evidence had been turned over to the FBI. It did not therefore have a copy of the tape. One was obtained, nevertheless, from Mary Ferrell, a critic who lived in the city of Dallas.

The committee then set out to find an acoustical consultant to analyze the tape. After consideration of five possible candidates, the committee picked the firm of Bolt, Beranek & Newman of Cambridge, Mass.

Bolt, Beranek & Newman can count among its many important forensic accomplishments an analysis of the tape-recorded sounds of the Kent State shooting incident in 1970 and the discovery and analysis of the 18-minute gap in the Watergate tapes.

B.B. & N. first analyzed the segment of the radio program, 'Four Days the Shocked the World', that had been believed to have covered the assassination. As it turned out, it was not contemporaneous with the actual shooting of the President.

The committee then forwarded the tape it had obtained from Mary Ferrell to B.B. & N., but no audible sounds could be discerned in the analysis.

Meanwhile, committee investigators working on the case in Dallas were in contact with Paul McCaghren, a retired assistant police chief who had been assigned to a special Dallas police assassination investigating squad.

McCaghren was one of several Dallas police veterans who donated their firsthand knowledge of the city to the committee. They 'read us into their backyard,' so to speak, as one of our investigators so aptly put it. Their help has been invaluable.

Among the original documents and tapes that McCaghren supplied the committee was a crucial November 22, 1963 dispatch tape along with the dictabelts that recorded the transmission from the motorcycle with the open mike. These materials were promptly sent to Bolt, Beranek & Newman.

To supplement the analysis of the tape, B.B. & N. experts also went to Dallas last month to conduct an acoustical reenactment based on the live firing of a rifle in Dealey Plaza.

In these tests, the Dallas Police Department was exceptionally cooperative. It obtained weapons, constructed the bullet 'traps' and rerouted traffic during the 5 hours of testing. Police marksmen fired rounds from the Book Depository, as well as from the 'grassy knoll.'

The final results of this work have only recently been received by the committee. Nevertheless, they have been thoroughly analyzed.

The man in charge of the Bolt, Beranek & Newman acoustical analysis is Dr. James E. Barger, the firm's chief scientist." [8]

In addition to Dr. Barger, the Committee selected Professors Mark Weiss and Ernest Aschkenasy of Queens College of the City University of New York to examine and confirm the experimental design, analysis, and conclusions of Bolt, Beranek & Newman (BBN).

In his testimony Dr. Barger described the process by which BBN acquired and analyzed the relevant data. A tape of the police recordings was made and a process known as adaptive filtering was applied to filter out the motorcycle noise in the sample. Acoustic events contained in the sample, such as the tolling of a bell and police dispatch activity were used to narrow down the window in which the shots were likely to occur. [9]

An experiment was set up in Dealey Plaza where recording microphones were placed 18 feet apart on Elm Street to simulate the location of a police motorcycle with an open microphone in the President's motorcade. Test shots were fired from the sixth floor of the Texas School Book Depository using a Mannlicher-Carcano rifle, both with the muzzle at the plane of the window, and with the muzzle two feet inside the window. Additional recordings were made using test shots fired from the grassy knoll using a Mannlicher-Carcano rifle and a pistol.

Dr. Barger explained to the Committee that when a gun shot is heard by a human observer or recorded by a microphone, it will consist of both a shock wave (created as the bullet passes through and rapidly displaces the air) and the actual sound of the muzzle blast. Echoes are then created as the resulting acoustic energy is reflected, scattered, and diffracted by objects in the environment.

For a rifle firing a supersonic bullet (travelling faster than the speed of sound), the shock wave will precede the muzzle blast (travelling at the speed of sound), and for a pistol firing a subsonic bullet, the muzzle blast will precede the shock wave. At any given point in an enclosed urban environment such as Dealey Plaza that has many large reflective surfaces, the pattern of acoustic energy presented to the ear of a listener, or to a microphone, will depend greatly on the location of the sound source and the location of the receiver, because these two factors will govern how the sound propagates, how it is reflected back, and how these two factors interact. Each combination of sound source, source location, and receiver location will generate a unique acoustic signature, similar to a fingerprint.

After the test firing, the sounds recorded by the various microphones on Elm Street were compared to the sounds on the Dallas Police motorcycle recording. The results showed that four impulse events at 137.70, 139.27, 145.15, and 145.61 seconds after the onset of the open microphone corresponded to Dealey Plaza test shots, and that the zone of maximum correlation moved down Elm Street over that time period (i.e. higher correlations were obtained with microphones positioned further down Elm Street toward the end of the time frame being examined).

This yielded a time span of 1.57 seconds between Shots 1 and 2, 5.88 seconds between Shots 2 and 3, and 0.46 seconds between Shots 3 and 4, for a total span of 7.91 seconds. The results indicated that Shot 3 was fired from the grassy knoll. Using computer simulation techniques Professors Weiss and Aschkenasy further refined the analysis and concluded with 95% certainty that a supersonic rifle shot was fired at President Kennedy from the grassy knoll.*

---

* The House Select Committee recommended that the Department of Justice examine the nature of the conspiracies to kill President Kennedy and Martin

Based on these data the House Select Committee on Assassinations concluded that two shooters had fired on the President, with one shot coming from the grassy knoll, but missing the President.

The Committee also examined Jack Ruby's extensive connections to organized crime, and, in the end, drew the following conclusions:

A. Lee Harvey Oswald fired three shots at President Kennedy. The second and third shots he fired struck the President. The third shot he fired killed the President.

1. President Kennedy was struck by two rifle shots fired from behind him.

2. The shots that struck President Kennedy from behind were fired from the sixth floor window of the southeast corner of the Texas School Book Depository.

3. Lee Harvey Oswald owned the rifle that was used to fire the shots from the sixth floor window of the southeast corner of the Texas School Book Depository building.

4. Lee Harvey Oswald, shortly before the assassination, had access to and was present on the sixth floor corner of the Texas School Book Depository building.

5. Lee Harvey Oswald's other actions tend to support the conclusion that he assassinated President Kennedy.

B. Scientific acoustical evidence establishes a high probability that two gunmen fired at President John F. Kennedy. Other scientific evidence does not preclude the possibility of two gunman firing at

---

Luther King. Instead the Department commissioned a study by the National Research Council, a branch of the National Academy of Sciences, which found that the BBN data and analysis did not support the conclusion of a shot from the grassy knoll with a 95% statistically significant probability. It was also determined that there was crosstalk between channels on the original dictabelt recording made by the Dallas Police Department. A subsequent study published by federal statistical expert D.B. Thomas found a 96% statistically significant probability for the grassy knoll gunman, and documented errors in the analyses used by both BBN and the NRC. [10, 11]

the President. Scientific evidence negates some specific conspiracy allegations.

C. The committee believes, on the basis of the evidence available to it, that President John F. Kennedy was probably assassinated as a result of a conspiracy. The committee is unable to identify the other gunman or the extent of the conspiracy.

  1. The committee believes, on the basis of the evidence available to it, that the Soviet Government was not involved in the assassination of President Kennedy.

  2. The committee believes, on the basis of the evidence available to it, that the Cuban Government was not involved in the assassination of President Kennedy.

  3. The committee believes, on the basis of the evidence available to it, that anti-Castro Cuban groups, as groups, were not involved in the assassination of President Kennedy, but that the available evidence does not preclude the possibility that individual members may have been involved.

  4. The committee believes, on the basis of the evidence available to it, that the national syndicate of organized crime, as a group, was not involved in the assassination of President Kennedy, but that the available evidence does not preclude the possibility that individual members may have been involved.

  5. The Secret Service, Federal Bureau of Investigation, and Central Intelligence Agency were not involved in the assassination of President Kennedy. [12]

CHAPTER 4

THE SEVEN BIG LIES OF THE MEDICAL EVIDENCE AND THE KENNEDY ASSASSINATION SMOKING GUN

German dictator Adolf Hitler discussed the Big Lie technique in his book *Mein Kampf*:

"…in the big lie there is always a certain force of credibility; because the broad masses of a nation are always more easily corrupted in the deeper strata of their emotional nature than consciously or voluntarily; and thus in the primitive simplicity of their minds they more readily fall victims to the big lie than the small lie, since they themselves often tell small lies in little matters but would be ashamed to resort to large-scale falsehoods. It would never come into their heads to fabricate colossal untruths, and they would not believe that others could have the impudence to distort the truth so infamously. Even though the facts which prove this to be so may be brought clearly to their minds, they will still doubt and waver and will continue to think that there may be some other explanation. For the grossly impudent lie always leaves traces behind it, even after it has been nailed down, a fact which is known to all expert liars in this world and to all who conspire together in the art of lying." [1]

Over a period of sixteen years the President's wounds were transformed from the facts officially recorded on November 22, 1963 into the completely

unrecognizable set of facts contained within the Report of the House Select
Committee on Assassinations (Figure 4-1), a transformation performed by

The Many Official Versions of President Kennedy's Wounds		
Date	Source	Wounds
11/22/1963	- Parkland hospital clinical treatment records - Autopsy records - FBI autopsy report	- small circular wound in the front of the neck - small circular wound at the base of the skull - small circular wound several inches down the back and two inches deep - large gaping hole in the upper right quadrant of the back of the head
11/24/1963	Autopsy report	same as Version 1, except that the wound in the back was also at the base of the neck, located where a buttoned dress collar would normally be positioned; the depth of the wound was not indicated.
9/24/1964	Warren Commission Report	same as Version 2, except that the back wound was definitely placed in the back of the neck and alleged to be the entrance point for a bullet that exited the front of the neck.
1/16/1969	Clark Panel Report	same as Version 3, except that the small circular wound previously at the base of the skull was repositioned to the top of the head.
3/29/1979	House Select Committee on Assassinations Report	- small circular wound in the front of the neck - small circular wound at the top of the skull; no damage to the back of the head - small circular wound several inches down the back, determined to be the entrance point for a bullet exiting the front of the neck - large gaping hole in the upper right quadrant of the front of the head

Figure 4-1. The five official versions of the President's wounds showing
their release dates and the source of the information.

employees and agents of the federal government with the goal of disguising the fact that the President was struck by more than two bullets. Since one shot missed the President and hit a bystander, three or more bullets striking the President meant four or more shots, decisively excluding the idea that Lee Harvey Oswald was the lone, unaided assassin of the President.

As of midnight November 22, 1963 it had been established by the Parkland Hospital doctors and the official autopsy that the President had: i) a shallow wound five inches down his back, ii) an entrance wound at the base of his skull, iii) a small wound in the front of his neck, and iv) a massive head wound that produced a large gaping hole in the back of his head (Figure 4-2, A and B).

By March 29, 1979 (the date the Select Committee report was officially submitted to the House of Representatives) the President's wounds had been transformed into: i) a matching set of entrance and exit wounds at the top of his head (Figure 4-2C), leaving the back of his head completely undisturbed, but resulting, despite autopsy photographs of the President's face to the contrary, in the complete obliteration of the right front of the President's skull, and ii) a matching set of entrance and exit wounds in the President's back and neck, which allegedly occurred because the President was leaning forward at a 45 degree angle between Zapruder Frames 188 and 226.

The Seven Big Lies that were deployed as the vehicle for this transformation have been hiding in plain sight for 50 years, and constitute the smoking gun of Kennedy assassination. These are:

1. By midnight of November 22, 1963 the President's autopsy had established that he had a shallow wound located five inches down his back and two inches to the right of his spinal column. Although the autopsy pathologists did not have access to the President's clothing, the wound's location corresponds exactly to the bullet holes in the President's shirt and suit jacket. This account is documented on the autopsy face sheet and in the written report of FBI agents Sibert and O'Neill. The next morning the chief autopsy pathologist, Dr. James Humes, spoke with Dr. Malcolm Perry of Parkland Hospital and learned that the President had a small wound in the front of his throat that had been obliterated by a tracheotomy. To explain this wound and accommodate the two bullet scenario, the autopsy pathologists repositioned the location of the back wound up into the President's neck in

their report of November 24, 1963, and claimed that the bullet had entered the back of the President's neck and exited the front. This false scenario was then presented as truth to the American public in the Warren Commission Report.

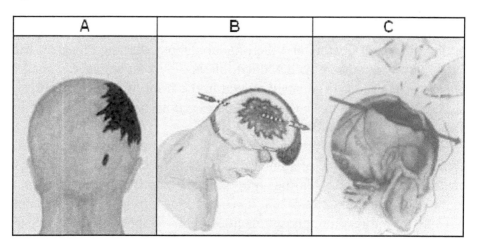

| A | B | C |

Figure 4-2. Warren Commission Exhibits 386 (A) and 388 (B) showing the Warren Commission's version of the "head shot", and (C) House Select Committee on Assassinations Exhibit F-66 showing the Committee's version. The Warren Commission scenario had the President facing the floor of his limousine when a bullet entered the base of his skull and exploded out of the top of his head. The Zapruder film instead shows that the President was sitting virtually upright (Figure 1-5B). The House Select Committee version had the bullet entering at the top of the President's head, but the autopsy found no entrance wound there, indicating that the scenario is a complete fabrication.

2. The House Select Committee on Assassinations found that the entrance wound the President's back was actually two inches lower than indicated in the Warren Commission Report. In order to accommodate the two bullet scenario, the Committee asserted that the President was leaning forward at a 45 degree angle, thus lowering the front of his neck relative to the back (Figure 3-5C). The Zapruder film shows the President sitting erect during the time he was shot in the back. The false assertion of a 45 degree forward-leaning posture was presented as truth to the American public in the House Select Committee on Assassinations report.

3. The autopsy pathologists found an entrance wound at the base of the President's skull, just above the occipital protuberance, and an inch to the right of the midline. The autopsy pathologists and the Warren Commission asserted that a bullet entered the base of the President's skull and exploded out of the top of his head because he was slumped over and facing the floor of his limousine. The Zapruder film shows that the President was not facing the floor of his limousine, and in fact was leaning forward at a slight angle (Figure 1-5). The false scenario that had the President facing the floor of his limousine at the time of the "head shot" was presented as truth to the American public in the Warren Commission Report.

4. The autopsy pathologists and the Warren Commission found an entrance wound that was located at the base of the President's skull. Based on photographs in the National Archives allegedly taken at the autopsy, the Clark Panel and House Select Committee on Assassinations asserted that the entrance wound was in fact four inches higher, at the top of the President's head. The House Select Committee forensic pathology panel insinuated that Dr. Humes, Senior Pathologist and Director of Laboratories at Bethesda Naval Hospital, Dr. Boswell, Chief of Pathology at Bethesda Naval Hospital, and Dr. Finck, Chief of the Wound Ballistics Pathology Branch of the Armed Forces Institute of Pathology, as well as the rest of the physicians, technical staff, and military commanders present, were all completely fooled into thinking that an extraneous piece of dried brain matter was a bullet hole in the President's skull. This is an assertion that is beyond reason or belief. Colonel Finck alone had studied over 400 autopsies involving gunshot wounds.[2] The wound was carefully inspected by Dr. Humes to determine if it was an entrance wound or an exit wound. In fact, in testimony before the House Select Committee Dr. Humes emphasized that he had examined "the President's skull from the inside when the brain was removed, with great care", leaving no doubt that there was only one entrance wound in the President's head, and that that wound was located at the base of the President's skull.[3] The false assertion that the President had an entrance wound at the top of his head was presented as truth to the American public by the Clark Panel and the House Select Committee on Assassinations.

5. The Parkland Hospital doctors all described a large gaping hole in the back of the President's head, with some stating the wound was so low that

cerebellar tissue was extruding from the wound. The official autopsy and the Warren Commission Report both documented a large head wound that extended well into the back of the President's head. In contrast to these official findings, the House Select Committee produced a photograph from the National Archives allegedly taken at the autopsy that not only showed the back of the President's head to be completely undamaged, it showed virtually every single hair to be perfectly in place. Either the Parkland doctors, the autopsy pathologists, the autopsy pathology staff, and the Warren Commission all hallucinated a large gaping hole in the back of the President's head, or the photograph is an obvious fraud.* The House Select Committee forensic pathology panel claimed to have reviewed the Warren Commission Report containing the statements of the Parkland doctors and the autopsy pathologists, yet no questions were asked about the discrepancy. The false assertion that the President had no damage to the back of his head was presented as truth to the American public by the House Select Committee on Assassinations.

6. The House Select Committee on Assassinations produced X-rays allegedly of the President showing the right front of the President's skull to be completely obliterated, yet autopsy photographs show the President's face to be completely intact and undamaged. The X-rays had been cropped to obscure the dental work. The X-rays and the autopsy photographs of the President's face are completely incompatible. Either the X-rays are false, or the photographs are false. Both cannot be true. Both were presented as truth to the American public by the House Select Committee on Assassinations.

7. The Warren Commission and Clark Panel both claimed that a single bullet entered the back of the President's neck, exited the front, and continued on to cause all of the injuries sustained by Governor Connally. This scenario ignores the fact that i) the President didn't have a wound in the back of his neck; the wound was five inches down his back, ii) in the Zapruder film Governor Connally displays no signs of injury until well after the President

* The morticians from Gawlers funeral home had to install a piece of rubber approximately 3.5 inches in diameter in the back of the President's head to prevent embalming fluid from leaking out. At the completion of their work the morticians felt that no damage to the President could be seen, and that an open casket funeral was possible. Curiously, the viewing and funeral were both closed casket. [4]

has been shot in the back, iii) the bullet is required to change direction for no apparent reason, iv) the recovered bullet is in pristine condition despite having struck several bones in Governor Connally, and v) the bullet shows no evidence of fragmentation despite allegedly having deposited numerous fragments in Governor Connally's body. The mass of the fragments plus the mass of the recovered bullet exceeds the mass of a single bullet. Although the single bullet theory is clearly impossible, it has been presented as truth to the American public for almost fifty years.

The Seven Big Lies were created by employees and agents of the federal government who stage-managed the process to conceal the fact that the President was struck by more than two bullets, which would invalidate any scenario that has Lee Harvey Oswald as the lone, unaided sniper. This leads to an inevitable conclusion:

President Kennedy was assassinated as the result of a conspiracy that emanated, wholly or in part, from within the federal government of the United States. There is no other reason why employees of the federal government would attempt to cover up such a massive crime.

CHAPTER 5

THE SEMINAL TEXTS

Over a thousand books have been written about the Kennedy assassination. Four of these, however, stand out as the seminal texts that have provided a foundation for understanding what actually happened on November 22, 1963. These are:

1. *Rush to Judgment* by Mark Lane (1966).

2. *Best Evidence: Disguise and Deception in the Assassination of President Kennedy* by David Lifton (1980).

3. *On the Trail of the Assassins* by Jim Garrison (1988).

4. *High Treason: The Assassination of President Kennedy - What Really Happened* by Robert Groden and Harrison Livingstone (1989).

RUSH TO JUDGMENT
BY MARK LANE

Mark Lane is a lawyer who was retained by the accused assassin's mother, Marguerite Oswald, to represent the interests of her son posthumously before the Warren Commission. This apparently so angered J. Edgar Hoover that he publicly declared that Lane's presence demonstrated that Marguerite Oswald was "emotionally unstable" and therefore an unreliable witness concerning the facts of the assassination, and in particular, facts that might indicate that her son was innocent.

Regardless of Oswald's actual guilt or innocence, Lane felt that all accused have the right to legal counsel, and he was disturbed by the fact that from the start, the Warren Commission presumed Oswald to be the lone assassin, and that its sole concern was to fill in the blanks around that central presumption of guilt.

To demonstrate this point, Lane presents the *modus operandi* of the Commission, as defined by its General Counsel, J. Lee Rankin. According to Rankin, the Commission would be divided into six areas of inquiry, each with its own senior and assistant attorneys:

1. Oswald's activities on November 22nd.

2. Oswald's background.

3. Oswald's career in the Marine Corps and his stay in the Soviet Union.

4. Oswald's murder in the Dallas police station.

5. Ruby's background.

6. The procedures employed to protect President Kennedy.

There was no panel, for example, to examine whether Oswald actually shot the President, or if there were additional shooters. From the outset, "Oswald the Lone Assassin" was the only scenario that would be considered, and, to this end, only evidence supporting "Oswald the Lone Assassin" would be favored, and all other evidence disfavored, or deliberately excluded.

Lane's book is essentially an indictment of the Warren Commission's failure to draw rational conclusions from the data that were assembled, in some cases drawing inferences that were diametrically opposed to the actual testimony received. It relies primarily on the report of the Commission itself, and how it squares with the 26 volumes of supporting testimony and exhibits from which it was allegedly derived. The book also includes supplementary taped testimony from significant witnesses.

From Lane's analysis, one gets the firm impression that "Oswald the Lone Assassin" was the Commission's sole *raison d'etre*.

In a chapter entitled "Where the Shots Came From", Lane examines the testimony and other evidence provided by numerous witnesses in Dealey Plaza. Of 90 witnesses asked where the shots came from, 58 stated that the shots came from the grassy knoll (Figures 5-1 through 5-6), with 32 believing

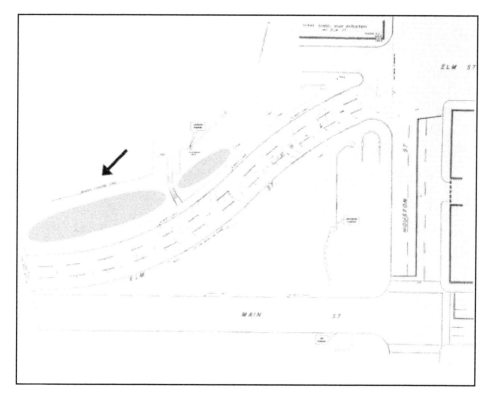

Figure 5-1. Portion of Warren Commission Exhibit 883, a schematic drawing of Dealey Plaza, modified to show the approximate location of the "grassy knoll", a strip of grass and trees on the north side of Elm Street. The term "shots from the grassy knoll" generally refers to shots fired from behind the fence overlooking the knoll (arrow). The Texas School Book Depository is at the top right.

they came from elsewhere. Of those 32, almost half were in the motorcade, and of those, almost all were government officials, their spouses, aides, or members of the local or federal police.

After the shots a swarm of police and others converged on the parking lot behind the grassy knoll (Figure 5-3). There are photographs of police climbing over the fence to get to the parking lot. In various home movies, people are seen running up the grassy knoll to see what happened. The parking lot behind the knoll soon became the central focus of police efforts to find the shooter. Dallas Police Chief Jesse Curry was recorded as ordering the police to

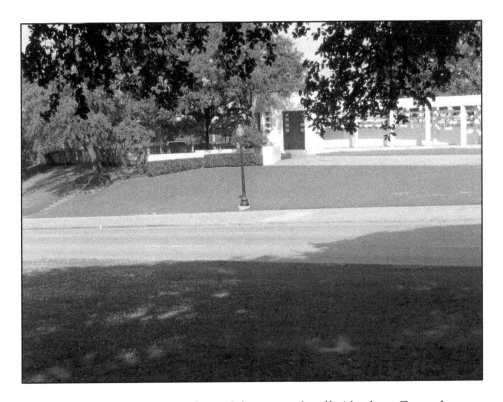

Figure 5-2. Contemporary view of the grassy knoll. Abraham Zapruder was standing on the pedestal at the center when he filmed the assassination. Note the picket fence at the left separating the knoll from the parking lot behind it. Most conspiracy theories assert that there was a sniper shooting over the fence at the President.

examine the top of the triple underpass adjacent to the knoll, and Sheriff J.E. Decker directed all available forces to converge on the parking lot to find the shooter. A police command post that was set up in that area was still active two hours after the shooting.

Yet the Commission concluded otherwise:

"…attention centered on the Texas School Book Depository Building as the source of the shots within a few minutes…No credible evidence suggests that the shots were fired from the railroad bridge over the Triple Underpass, the nearby railroad yards or any place other than the Texas School Book Depository Building…In contrast

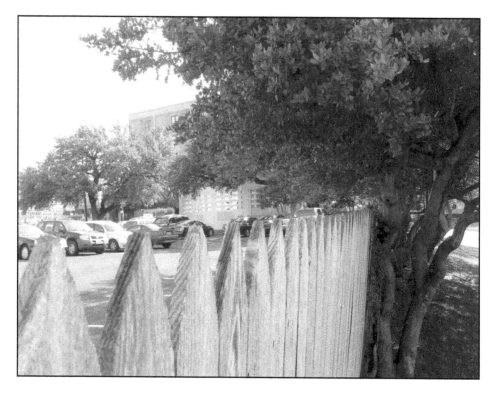

Figure 5-3. Contemporary view of the parking lot behind the grassy knoll. The railroad tower occupied by Lee Bowers stood at the edge of the parking lot, with Bowers facing the fence at the time of the assassination. CIA spy E. Howard Hunt is alleged to have been apprehended in the train yard behind the parking lot shortly after the assassination (Figure 5-7; Chapter 8).

to the testimony of the witnesses who heard and observed shots fired from the Depository, the Commission's investigation has disclosed no credible evidence that any shots were fired from anywhere else."

Lane goes on to examine the observations of Lee Bowers, Jr., whose testimony provides a stark example of how Commission functionaries tailored witness testimony to produce the "Oswald the Lone Assassin" conclusion.

Bowers worked as a railroad towerman for the Union Terminal Company, occupying a 14 foot tower that overlooked the railroad yard and parking lot just behind the grassy knoll. He sat facing the assassination site. He testified

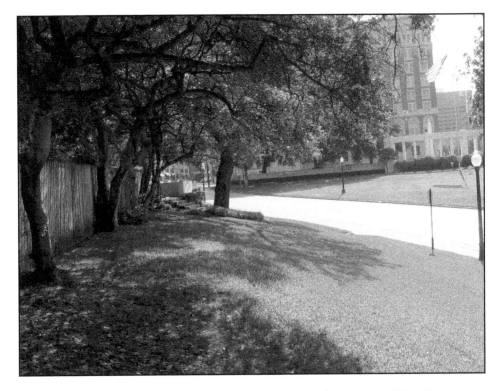

Figure 5-4. Contemporary view from the grassy knoll onto Elm Street.

that he saw two men standing behind the fence above the knoll just before the assassination, and that these were the only strangers in the area who were not railroad personnel. When the shots were fired the two men were still there.

The following exchange occurred with the Commission:

Bowers: Something occurred in this particular spot which was out of the ordinary, which attracted my eye for some reason, which I could not identify.

Commission: You couldn't describe it?

Bowers: Nothing that I could pinpoint as having happened that –

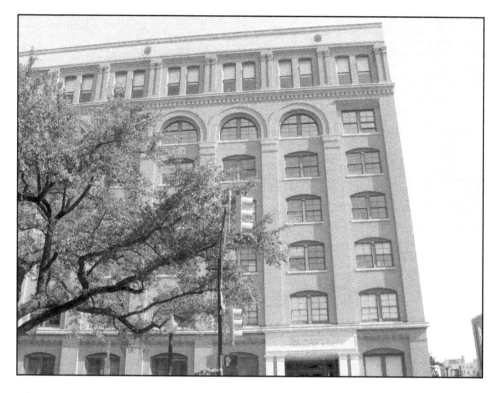

Figure 5-5. Contemporary view of the former Dallas School Book Depository, now called the Dallas County Administration Building. The sniper's nest is on the right on the sixth floor.

At this point Bowers was cut off by Commission counsel and asked an unrelated question. Lane subsequently conducted a filmed and tape recorded interview with Bowers and asked him to elaborate on this critical point:

Bowers: At the time of the shooting, in the vicinity of where the two men I have described were, there was a flash of light or, as far as I am concerned, something I could not identify, but there was something that occurred which caught my eye in this immediate area of the embankment. Now, what this was, I could not state at that time and at this time I could not identify it, other than there was some unusual occurrence – a flash of light or smoke or something which caused me to feel like something out of the ordinary had occurred there.

76

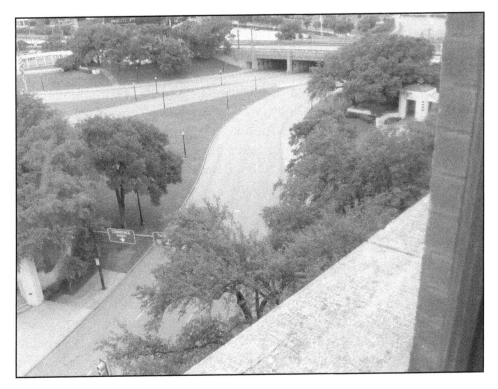

Figure 5-6. Contemporary view of Elm Street from the sixth floor of the Texas School Book Depository. The grassy knoll is at the right. The lower 'X' in the street at the center marks the location where President Kennedy was hit in the back; the upper 'X' marks the location of the so-called "head shot".

Lane: In reading your testimony, Mr. Bowers, it appears that just as you were about to make that statement, you were interrupted in the middle of the sentence by the Commission counsel, who then went into another area.

Bowers: Well, that's correct. I mean I was simply trying to answer his questions, and he seemed to be satisfied with the answer to that one and did not care for me to elaborate.

Several railroad employees standing on the railroad bridge over Elm Street thought that the shots came from the bushes and trees to their immediate left at the crest of the knoll, and they observed a puff of smoke six to eight feet above the ground. Patrolman J.M. Smith told *The Texas Observer* that he smelled gunpowder, and yet when called before the Commission he was not asked any questions about the smell of gunpowder behind the fence.

Senator Ralph Yarborough, riding in the third car of the motorcade with Vice President Lyndon Johnson, also told *The Texas Observer* that he smelled the strong and persistent odor of gunpowder when passing the knoll. Senator Yarborough was not called before the Commission.

After the assassination Oswald left the Book Depository for his rooming house. There are two versions of how he got there. The Commission maintains that Oswald walked seven blocks, took a bus ride back toward the Depository, walked some more, took a taxi ride past his rooming house to the 500 block of North Beckley Avenue, walked a further 700 yards back to his rooming house, changed and retrieved his gun, and then walked a mile to the corner of East 10th Street and Patton Avenue, where he murdered Dallas Patrol Officer J.D. Tippit, all in a span of less than 43 minutes.*

The Dallas police produced a bus transfer receipt and the Commission heard testimony from bus driver Cecil McWatters, who the police allege made a positive identification of Oswald in a lineup. Yet when the Commission asked McWatters if he could identify Oswald as the man who had boarded his bus, he stated that he could not, and that at the police lineup:

"...I told them (the Dallas police) that there was one man in the lineup was about the size and the height and complexion of a man that got on my bus, but as far as positively identifying the man I could not do it."

The Commission ignored the testimony of Deputy Sheriff Roger Craig, who stated that approximately 15 minutes after the assassination he heard someone whistling loudly near the corner of Elm and Houston, and turned to see Oswald running toward and entering a light colored Nash Rambler station wagon driven by a dark complexioned male. Early in the evening of November 22nd Craig went to the office of Captain Will Fritz, where Oswald

---

* It is interesting to note that in the Commission's version Oswald went past his rooming house and exited the cab approximately midway between his rooming house and Jack Ruby's residence.

was being interrogated, and confirmed that Oswald was the man that he had seen running toward the station wagon. Captain Fritz then asked Oswald, "What about this station wagon?", to which Oswald replied, "That station wagon belongs to Mrs. Paine. Don't try to tie her into this. She had nothing to do with it." *

Lane also relates a strange incident that occurred just after Oswald arrived at his rooming house. The housekeeper, Earlene Roberts, said that shortly after Oswald arrived, a police car drove up to the house and parked outside.

Commission: Where was it parked?

Roberts: It was parked in front of the house...

Commission: Did this police car stop directly in front of your house?

Roberts: Yes - it stopped directly in front of my house...

Commission: Where was Oswald when this happened?

Roberts: In his room...

Commission: Were there two uniformed policemen in the car?

Roberts: Oh, yes.

Commission: And one of the officers sounded the horn?

Roberts: Just kind if 'tit-tit' twice.**

---

* Oswald's wife and children were living with Mrs. Ruth Paine in nearby Irving, and she owned a light colored Nash Rambler station wagon. Ruth Paine had secured the job for Oswald at the Texas School Book Depository.
** Patrol Officer J.D. Tippit's car was found with a spare uniform hanging in the window. However, Roberts told investigators that the car that she observed bore identification number 207. According to Warren Commission Exhibit 2645, on November 22, 1963 car number 207 was assigned to

Lane goes on to describe the hunt for Oswald, and the strange case of Officer J.D. Tippit's demise.

About 15 minutes after the shooting Dallas police broadcast a description of the wanted man: "a slender white male about thirty, five feet ten, one sixty five". Accounts differ as to how the police came upon this information so quickly, but the hunt was nonetheless on.

At 12:44 all police cars were told to report to Dealey Plaza. One minute later Tippit and another officer were told to "move into the Central Oak Cliff area". At 12:54 the dispatcher spoke with Tippit and verified that he was in Oak Cliff. At 1:08 Tippit tried to call dispatch twice, but was unsuccessful, and he was subsequently shot to death with four bullets.

Discrepancies between the original Dallas police logs and the comparable FBI transcripts hint at strange occurrences that afternoon.

The original Dallas police log shows that Tippit's assigned call number was 78, and indicates that both of his final calls were not answered. The FBI transcript of the exact same recording shows different, unassigned call numbers substituted for Tippit's number, and indicates that the calls were answered, but were garbled.

The Dallas version shows that Tippit tried to call twice, but that no one spoke with him, and the FBI version, used by the Warren Commission, shows that no such calls by Tippit ever existed because the calls had been assigned to other call numbers, not Tippit's.

In any event, Officer Tippit was shot dead next to his patrol car. Witness accounts vary as to what actually happened. Some witnesses describe a single shooter resembling Oswald, others a single shooter who was short and heavy with bushy hair, and another witness said that there were two shooters, with one gunman being short and heavy, and his accomplice described as tall and thin with light khaki trousers and a white shirt.

Adding to the uncertainty surrounding Officer Tippit's death was the finding that the four bullets extracted from his body consisted of two

---

Patrol Officer J.M. Valentine. Valentine stated that he went to the Texas School Book Depository at 12:45 PM, parking his car at the curb. He was assigned to the fifth floor and remained there until about 4 PM. The Warren Commission Report also notes a connection between Earlene Roberts and Jack Ruby. Roberts' sister, Bertha Cheek, met with Jack Ruby four days before the assassination to offer him financial support for a new club. [1]

different types of ammunition, suggesting that two different guns may have been used.

Tippet himself may have known Jack Ruby. Ruby's appearance at the epicenter of the assassination is one of the more curious aspects of the Kennedy tragedy - Ruby was connected to the assassination in a number of ways beyond Oswald's murder, and, in fact, also seems to have been associated with Officer Tippit.

Greeting President Kennedy on his arrival in Dallas was an advertisement in *The Dallas Morning News* suggesting that Kennedy was in league with Communists in Moscow. The signer of that advertisement was Bernard Weissman, an avowed anti-Communist, who stated before the Commission that the funds for the advertisement were raised by Joseph P. Grinnan, a member of the John Birch Society, a right wing opponent of Communism.

Lane relates how he gave the Commission information concerning a two hour meeting involving Weissman, Tippit and Ruby on November 14, 1963 at the Carousel Club. The allegations came from an informant for Thayer Waldo, a reporter with the *Fort Worth Star Telegram*. The informant told Waldo that he saw Ruby sit down at a table with Tippit and Weissman, and that the three men were still having a serious discussion two hours later when he left the club. The informant came to fear for his life after the assassination. Waldo was questioned by Commission counsel, but was not asked about the meeting. Ruby's bartender Larry Crafard later told the FBI that Weissman had been in the Carousel a number of times, and that Ruby had specifically referred to him by name.

The *New York Herald Tribune* reported on December 5, 1963 that Eva Grant, Ruby's sister, said in a telephone interview that both she and Ruby knew Tippit, and that "Tippit used to come into the Vegas Club and Carousel Club", and that her brother "called him buddy". Testifying before Commission counsel, Grant stated that "Tippit was in our club sometime a month previous to this – previous to his killing." At least six witnesses, including Dallas Police Lieutenant George C. Arnett, confirmed that Ruby knew Tippit.

The Commission conclusion: it could find no credible evidence that Ruby was acquainted with Tippit.

In fact, Ruby knew many, if not most, of the members of the Dallas Police Department, due in good measure to the carnal largesse he generously provided as operator of the Carousel Club. In a chapter entitled "A Friend of the Dallas Police" Lane catalogs the many ways in which Jack Ruby ingratiated himself with the Dallas Police. When police officers visited the Carousel they were admitted free of charge and given free drinks and meals. In some cases access to strippers was provided. Carousel staff testified that Ruby was on a first name basis with many of the officers in the department. Hugh Smith, a former Dallas police officer, stated that a fellow Dallas police officer had "used Ruby's apartment on several occasions". Benny Bickers, owner of a club adjacent to the Carousel, said that it was common knowledge that Ruby was at the Dallas Police Department almost every day. One part time employee, Richard Proeber, told the FBI that there "was talk amongst Ruby's help that Ruby was 'paying off' the Dallas Police Department for special favors."

Perhaps the most telling account of Jack Ruby's influence on the Dallas Police was provided to the Commission by Nancy Perrin Rich. Rich arrived in Dallas in May 1962, searching for her missing husband, Robert Perrin, who had a history of gunrunning during the Spanish Civil War. When she arrived in town she was shown extraordinary hospitality by the Dallas Police, and was eventually introduced to Jack Ruby, who offered her a job as a bartender at the Carousel. She told the Commission, "I don't think there is a cop in Dallas that doesn't know Jack Ruby. He practically lived at that station. They lived in his place. Even the lowest patrolman on the beat."

Ruby eventually beat her at work, and she went to the Police Department to file a complaint. She relates that she "was refused", and that she "was told if I did that I would never win it and get myself in more trouble than I bargained for." She was later arrested twice, and released with the advice that she not bring charges against Ruby.

That account, however, is overshadowed by what she subsequently told the Commission about Ruby. She testified to a meeting that included herself, a lieutenant colonel from the military, her husband, and an individual named Dave Cherry, who worked as a bartender at the University Club in Dallas. At the meeting Cherry and the colonel offered Robert Perrin $10,000 to bring refugees out of Cuba and into Miami. To Nancy Rich that amount seemed excessive for the services that were to be provided.

She described a second meeting that included herself, the colonel, this time in uniform, her husband, Cherry, and several others, some of whom appeared to be Cuban or Latin. At that meeting the terms of their proposed assignment were expanded to include running military hardware into Cuba,

82

then bringing refugees out. Rich requested $25,000. At this point, "A knock comes on the door and who walks in but my little friend Jack Ruby." Rich states that it appeared to her that Ruby had brought a large amount of cash with him, disappeared into another room with the colonel, and then left. Eventually the colonel raised the offer to $15,000, which was declined.

Lane subsequently spoke with Rich about the testimony she gave to the Commission concerning the second meeting, and he documents how unpleasant facts were omitted from the record. Rich told Lane that she had reviewed her testimony before the Commission, and that in fact she had "told Mr. Hubert and Mr. Griffin that in the apartment building, in a little storeroom outside of the apartment building, out in back, was a cache of military armaments" that included automatic rifles, land mines, and twenty to thirty cases of hand grenades, but that the Commission "chose to discount it... I can attest to the fact that at the time it was given it was told to be stricken from the record...I didn't think there would be (any record of it), considering Mr. Griffin said, 'Strike that from the record'."

Lane's analysis shows that Ruby's relationship to the assassination is complex and multifaceted. Despite his obvious connections to organized crime, he not only knew and successfully manipulated the Dallas Police Department and judicial system, he also served as paymaster for efforts to remove Castro, thus bringing him into the orbit of the CIA as one of the financial connection points between the Mafia, the CIA, and Cuban affairs.

Lane further documents numerous instances in which the FBI and Commission bullied, cajoled, and threatened witnesses if they did not offer the desired testimony. Dean Andrews was a New Orleans attorney who had been consulted by Oswald concerning modification of Oswald's Marine Corps discharge. Immediately after the assassination, Andrews was contacted to represent Oswald by an individual who identified himself as Clay Bertrand. The FBI insisted that Bertrand existed only in Andrews' imagination. According to Lane, the FBI closed the file on Andrews by writing that Andrews agreed that Bertrand never existed, yet when Andrews appeared before the Commission he stated that he had never made such a statement to the FBI, and in fact had recently seen Bertrand.

Patrick Dean was a sergeant in the Dallas Police Department who had interrogated Jack Ruby after Oswald was shot. Dean was interviewed by Commission counsel Burt Griffin, and he told Griffin that Ruby had stated that he had "planned to kill Oswald two nights prior" and that Ruby had entered the Police Department basement by simply walking down the Main Street ramp. At one point Griffin dismissed the court reporter and spoke to Dean off the record. Griffin told Dean that "there were particular things in there that were not true", and, in fact, "Jack Ruby didn't tell you that he entered the basement via the Main Street ramp", and that "Jack Ruby did not tell you that he had thought or planned to kill Oswald two nights prior."

Lane's book clearly demonstrates that the singular purpose of the Warren Commission was not to determine who killed Kennedy, but rather to distort the facts and create an elaborate web of lies to promote, from the outset, the "Oswald the Lone Assassin" scenario. Lane describes how one of the Commission members, Gerald Ford, provided further insight on this point in his book, *Portrait of an Assassin*:

"No sooner had the Commission investigating President Kennedy's assassination assembled its staff and tentatively outlined methods of operation than it was plunged into an astounding problem. On Wednesday, January 22, the members of the Commission were hurriedly called into emergency session by the chairman. Mr. J. Lee Rankin, newly appointed General Counsel for the Commission, had received a telephone call from Texas. The caller was Mr. Waggoner Carr, the Attorney General of Texas. The information was that the FBI had an 'undercover agent' and that that agent was none other than Lee Harvey Oswald, the alleged assassin of President Kennedy!

Prior to that day the newspapers had carried an inconspicuous article or two speculating on whether Oswald could have been an agent of any United States Government agency. Mrs. Marguerite Oswald had made statements that she thought her son must have been tied in with the CIA or the State Department. But now the alarm had been sounded by a high official; and the Dallas prosecutor, Mr. Henry Wade, who had also reported the rumor, was himself a former FBI man...

...The Texas officials slipped into the nation's capital with complete anonymity. They met with Lee Rankin and other members of the staff and told what they knew. The information was that Lee Oswald was actually hired by the FBI; that he was assigned undercover-agent number 179; that he was on the FBI payroll at two hundred dollars a month starting in September 1962 and that he was still on their payroll the day he was apprehended in the Texas Theatre after having gunned down Officer J.D. Tippit!"

In his book Ford stated that the Commission had two sets of responsibilities: first, to ascertain, evaluate, and report the facts, and second, to serve the national interests – to insure that no disunity resulted and that American institutions remained intact. Commission General Counsel J. Lee Rankin put it more succinctly: "We do have a dirty rumor that is very bad for the Commission, the problem, and it is very damaging to the agencies that are involved in it and it must be wiped out insofar as it is possible to do so by this Commission."

BEST EVIDENCE
BY DAVID LIFTON

In 1966 David Lifton was a graduate student in engineering at UCLA. While there he became entangled in an ongoing debate with Law School Professor Wesley Liebeler, a former Assistant Counsel for the Warren Commission, concerning the Kennedy assassination. In June 1966 Lifton wrote a 30,000 word article for *Ramparts* magazine entitled "The Case for Three Assassins". Lifton's research led him to publish a book entitled *Best Evidence: Disguise and Deception in the Assassination of John F. Kennedy* in 1980, focusing attention on the Kennedy autopsy and the strange events surrounding it.

His book opens in October 1966 with a conversation that he had with Liebeler in which Lifton maintained that a bullet was removed from the President's head, citing the report by FBI agents Sibert and O'Neill that mentioned "surgery of the head area, namely, in the top of the skull". Liebeler then composed a memorandum to Chief Justice Warren, Attorney General Ramsey Clark, Kennedy family attorney Burke Marshall, and all of the former Warren Commissioners. In the memo he indicated that although no surgery had been performed on the President's head at the hospital, information about the President's stated head surgery that was observed at autopsy did not appear in the Warren Commission Report or 26 volumes of Testimony and Exhibits.

Lifton had hoped in vain that the Warren Commission inquiry would be re-opened.

Lifton describes visiting New York during a recess at UCLA graduate school and seeing a presentation by Mark Lane in September 1964. At that time he found that a conspiracy was hard to believe because too many people would have had to have been involved. He nonetheless found Lane's presentation convincing, particularly questions about how the throat wound had undergone a transformation from entrance wound at Parkland to exit wound in Bethesda. He became fascinated by the assassination, particularly the medical and technical aspects.

His initial focus was to examine a significant anomaly observed in the Zapruder film, as presented in Warren Commission Volume 18. The problem was that the two frames following the "head shot" were reversed, falsely giving President Kennedy the appearance of initially moving forward after being struck, when in fact his head was rocketed backward and to the left. Lifton wrote to FBI Director J. Edgar Hoover concerning the problem, and he received a reply acknowledging the error. Hoover stated that it was due to a "printing error".

Lifton begins to interview witnesses, and he becomes adept at extracting crucial information in an unbiased manner. Eventually he comes to focus on the medical evidence, and delves into learning the basic elements of neuroanatomy and standard autopsy procedure, both of which are described in detail in his book.

Lifton later confronts Liebeler again about the "surgery of the head area, namely, in the top of the skull" remark noted in the FBI reports on the autopsy, as well as testimony by Commander Humes contained in Volume 2 of the Warren Commission Report, in which a parasagital laceration and bisection of the corpus callosum (the large band of fibers deep within the brain connecting the left and right hemispheres) are described. Liebeler contacts a pathologist friend and describes the wounds over the phone, not letting on that he is describing the autopsied brain of the President of the United States. The pathologist states that it sounded as if the deceased "was hit by an axe".

Based on the Bethesda pathologists' observation that the President had surgery of the skull, Lifton comes to believe that the body of the President may have been intercepted in transit and modified so as to achieve a predetermined outcome, i.e. that the President had been hit by only two bullets, both shot from behind, and that one of these bullets also caused all of the injuries observed in Governor Connally.

Lifton then focuses on the condition of the body when it left Parkland Hospital compared to its condition on arrival at the Bethesda morgue. The FBI agents at the autopsy reported that "the complete body was wrapped in a sheet and the head area contained an additional wrapping which was saturated with blood."

Lifton comes to believe that there are two time periods in which the President's body could have been diverted and altered: i) during the trip from Dallas to Washington on Air Force One, or ii) the period between the arrival of the ambulance at the front of Bethesda Naval Hospital and the start of the autopsy. He notes that the ambulance containing the casket arrived at the hospital at 6:55 PM, the body was received for autopsy at 7:35 PM, and that the autopsy began at 8:00 PM, after pictures and X-rays were taken. There was therefore a period of an hour and five minutes between when the casket arrived and when the autopsy began.

Of special note is the fact that FBI Agents Sibert and O'Neill were ordered to leave the examination room during the period when the pictures and X-rays were taken. Lifton again consults the report of FBI agents Sibert and O'Neill for a first hand account:

"On arrival at the Medical Center, the ambulance stopped in front of the main entrance, at which time Mrs. Jacqueline Kennedy and Attorney General Robert Kennedy embarked from the ambulance and entered the building. The ambulance was thereafter driven around to the rear entrance where the President's body was removed and taken into an autopsy room. Bureau Agents assisted in the moving of the casket to the autopsy room. A tight security was immediately placed around the autopsy room by the Naval facility and the U.S. Secret Service. Bureau Agents made contact with Mr. Roy Kellerman, the Assistant Secret Service Agent in Charge of the White House Detail, and advised him of the Bureau's interest in this matter."

Lifton paints a picture of utter confusion in front of the Bethesda Medical Center. He interviews top military officials who were at the scene for their recollections, and consults the *Dallas Morning News* to obtain a list of the names and home towns of the seven military men who were assigned to the casket team and who escorted the President's body from the time it arrived at Andrews Air Force Base to the grave site on Monday, November 25th.

He sets out to interview the members of the team:

1. Marine Lance Corporal Timothy Cheek remembered that the helicopter that transported them arrived well in advance of the ambulance bearing the President's body. They went to the front of the Medical Center where the body was supposed to be, got out of their truck, then got back into the truck because the body wasn't there. The officer in charge, Army 1st Lieutenant Samuel R. Bird, along with General Phillip Wehle, determined that the body was gone, so the team went to the other entrance, at the morgue, where they milled around and eventually located the body at the morgue door. Cheek reported that no FBI men were present when the ambulance was unloaded, with six of their team present to do the unloading. This contrasts with Sibert and O'Neill's account that the FBI Agents helped to unload the casket, with no mention of the presence of the casket team. Cheek noticed that the casket was damaged, with one handle completely broken off. In his book *Death of a President* William Manchester mentioned that damage to the casket occurred when it was unloaded from the undertaker's hearse onto the plane. Cheek tells Lifton that Lieutenant Bird had written a report and distributed a copy to each of his men. Cheek sends Lifton a copy.

2. Army Sergeant James L. Felder remembered a more complicated situation in which two ambulances were deployed, one to carry the Kennedys and the President's body, the other to serve as a decoy due to the large crowd that had assembled. The team was informed of this strategy. The first ambulance pulled up to the hospital, the Kennedys got out, and the ambulance then pulled away. The team attempted to follow the ambulance but was unsuccessful. The team returned to the front of the hospital, where a second ambulance was waiting. Felder said at one point there were two ambulances in front of the hospital and it was confusing as to which one had the body. The team eventually went to the back of the hospital, found the ambulance with the casket and unloaded it. Felder did not remember FBI agents unloading the casket from the ambulance.

3.   Another member of the casket team, **Navy SA Hubert Clark**, independently verified the presence of a decoy ambulance at Bethesda. Clark mentioned that no FBI men were present at the transfer of the casket from the ambulance, but that General Godfrey McHugh, a friend of the Kennedy family, had moved one of the pallbearers aside to lay his hands on the casket.

4. **Air Force Staff Sergeant Richard Gaudreau** reported a vague recollection of a second ambulance, while recalling a general picture of confusion as to where to go that night.

5.   When **Coast Guard Yeoman George Barnum** reported back for duty after the funeral, his superior officer at Coast Guard Headquarters told him to write a report, which he retained, primarily for the historical interest of his children. His account is similar to the others, namely that the Kennedys got out of the ambulance containing the casket, the team then tried to follow the ambulance, lost sight of it, and went to the back of the morgue only to find that the ambulance was not there, and eventually they found and unloaded the casket from the ambulance. He attributed much of the confusion to the large crowds that were present at the Medical Center.

    In August 1979 Lifton interviewed General Wehle's aide, Richard Lipsey, who had been mentioned in the Report of the House Select Committee on Assassinations. Lipsey stated that there were two ambulances that night. The first was at the front of the motorcade and contained Jacqueline Kennedy, and the second was much further back. He was told that the President's body was in the second ambulance. Lipsey believed that the plan had been formulated by the White House to allow the second ambulance to go directly to the back of the hospital. Lifton mentioned that Jacqueline Kennedy had been riding in the ambulance that contained the casket, and Lipsey responded that his perception was based on what he had been told at a meeting at Andrews Air Force Base before Air Force One had landed.

    Lifton also interviewed J.S. Layton Ledbetter, Chief of the Day at

Bethesda, who verified that there were two ambulances that arrived in the same motorcade, and that the ambulance carrying the President's body had quietly entered the morgue area in the back of the hospital, largely unobserved.

Lifton begins to speculate as to what might have happened at Bethesda between 7:10 PM and 8:00 PM. The casket team, confused by the two ambulances, eventually found an ambulance with the casket, and carried the casket into the morgue at 8:00 PM. The body, however, was already inside the morgue, having been escorted in by FBI Agents Sibert and O'Neill.

In an interview with Warren Commission Assistant Counsel Arlen Specter on March 12, 1964, Sibert and O'Neill indicated that the time of the preparation for the autopsy was 7:17 PM.

Lifton files a Freedom of Information request with the Military District of Washington for all documents pertaining to the handling of the President's body. He receives an attachment to a report by Colonel Phillipe P. Boas, the Provost Marshal:

"At about 1914 hours (7:14 PM) the CG [Commanding General] arrived with his Aide. I was informed by the General to remain with him and that he would subsequently advise me as to the details of my responsibility for subsequent action. At about this time the postmortem examination of the remains was initiated."

All of this presents an eerily strange picture of the autopsy preliminaries beginning about 7:15 PM, with the body already in the morgue, yet the casket team arriving and carrying in the casket 45 minutes later at 8:00 PM.

Lifton interviews members of the Bethesda staff who were present at the autopsy:

1. John Stringer was the autopsy photographer. He said that he helped lift the President out of the coffin. He did not see any member of the casket team. Lifton asked if he took photographs of the right lung, which had shown distinct bruising, and he replied that such pictures had been taken. Lifton knew that there were no pictures of the right lung in the collection at the National Archives and that the total number of pictures in the collection agreed with the number reported by Sibert and O'Neill, suggesting that some pictures had been removed and others added. Lifton asks about the location of the damage:

Lifton: When you lifted him out, was the main damage to the skull on the top or in the back?

Stringer: In the back.

Lifton: In the back?…High in the back or lower in the back?

Stringer: In the occipital, in the neck there, up above the neck.

Lifton: In other words, the main part of his head that was blasted away was in the occipital part of the skull?

Stringer: Yes, in the back part.

2. Lieutenant Commander Dennis Duane David was Chief of the Day for the Medical School on November 22, 1963. He said that he knew that the casket in the official motorcade was empty. The first ambulance to arrive had the President's body; the second ambulance had an empty casket that was unloaded by the ceremonial casket team. He mentioned that he was told by Dr. Boswell, one of the three autopsy pathologists, that there were two caskets and that the second one was empty. The first ambulance with the President's body arrived before the Kennedys had arrived in front, and it had six or seven men, who he presumed to be Secret Service agents, in back with the casket. He said that the casket was in a black Cadillac ambulance that resembled a hearse, distinctly different from the standard gray Navy ambulance. He stated that the black Cadillac ambulance arrived with the body fifteen to thirty minutes before the arrival of the motorcade in front of the medical center, and that he personally viewed Mrs. Kennedy get out of the ambulance, which contained the Dallas casket that was apparently empty. He noted that the first casket with the President's body was a plain metal casket that was gray, not the polished bronze casket used in Dallas.

3. At the time of the assassination **Paul Kelly O'Connor** was in Bethesda's laboratory school studying to become a medical technologist. He was on duty the night of the assassination and assisted the pathologists in the President's autopsy. He said that the body arrived at exactly 8 PM in a cheap gray shipping casket, not the ornate bronze ceremonial casket into which the President's body was placed in Dallas, and that the body was contained in a standard rubber body bag with a zipper on it that went from head to toe. O'Connor stated that he was certain that the time was 8 PM, because it was he who had logged the time in the official log book. He further stated that the large head wound was in the occipital-parietal area and extended into the frontal area of the brain. He estimated its dimensions to be about four by eight inches, and he thought that most of the President's brain was missing. O'Connor also thought that the body had arrived at Bethesda by helicopter. Lifton concludes that O'Connor may have been mistaken about the body's arrival time because he also said that the body left the morgue at 5:30 AM the next morning, while the casket team record shows a 4:00 AM departure.*

4. James Curtis Jenkins worked as a laboratory technician at Bethesda and was present at the autopsy. He recalled that the President arrived in a plain, simple casket, "not something you'd expect a President to be in". Jenkins observed a large wound in the back of the President's head and concluded that the President had been shot from the front. He was very surprised with the official conclusion that the President had been shot in the head from the back. He spoke of men in civilian clothes who seemed to be directing the autopsy, and who exhibited an attitude of animosity toward Dr. Humes, Dr. Boswell, and Dr. Finck. Lifton mentioned that in the official record there were only five men at the autopsy in civilian

---

* Lifton later confirmed with Aubrey Rike, one of two Dallas funeral home employees who put the body in the bronze casket, that a body bag was not used. According to Rike, the President's body was put on a plastic liner, thought to have come from a mattress cover, to keep blood away from the interior satin lining of the casket. He emphatically denied that a body bag was used.

clothes – FBI Agents Sibert and O'Neill, and Secret Service Agents Kellerman, Greer, and O'Leary – and Jenkins insisted that there were many more there, sitting in the gallery. He stated that these men seemed to be trying to convince Dr. Humes that the back wound extended through to the front of the body, although at the time the autopsy team had no knowledge of the wound in the President's neck. After the internal organs had been removed, Jenkins observed the doctors probing the back wound, and from the front he could see the probe making an indentation on the pleura, pushing the skin up. There had obviously been no entrance into the chest cavity, and he described the location of the wound as being low in the chest, at the level of the bronchus of the lungs (the point at which the windpipe splits into left and right branches). When Lifton informs Jenkins that the autopsy photographs show the back of the President's head to be intact, he replies "…there's no possible way…It's not possible."

5. Edward Reed was an X-ray technician at the Bethesda autopsy. He thought that the President's head wound was more posterior than anterior, and he formed the opinion that the President had been shot from the front.

6. Jerrol Custer was another X-ray technician at the Bethesda autopsy. He said that the head wound was enormous, and that he believed that the President had been shot from the front, based on his hunting experience. He said that he had exposed X-rays showing the back of the President's head had been blown off. The X-rays were taken at the morgue and to develop them he had to pass through the hospital lobby with a Secret Service escort to the upper floors of the facility. On the second or third trip he saw Jacqueline Kennedy arrive at the main entrance, and he passed her in the lobby with an armload of film. To Lifton, this is the clearest evidence that the ambulance that transported the Kennedys from the airport to the medical center contained an empty casket, because the President's autopsy was well under way when that ambulance arrived.

7. Floyd Albert Reibe was a student of the School of Medical Photography at the U.S. Navy Medical School at the time of the assassination, and was the duty photographer that night. He describes the casket in which the body arrived as being a shipping casket, in which the whole lid could be removed after taking off some thumbscrews. He had a vague recollection of the body being in a dark body bag with zippers. He described taking pictures, such as one of the President's back wound while he was laying on his stomach, that Lifton recognized as not being in the collection at the National Archives.

It's clear from the interviews and testimony assembled by Lifton that the bronze ornamental casket unloaded off of Air Force One did not contain the body of the President. By the time the ambulance transporting that casket and the Kennedys arrived at Bethesda Medical Center, the body of the President was already on the autopsy table and the autopsy was well under way.

Lifton attempts to pinpoint the time and place where the transfer could have occurred, and ultimately comes to speculate on the possibility that it could have happened aboard Air Force One, particularly during the time frame when Lyndon Johnson took the oath of office.

In all likelihood America will never know with certainty.

ON THE TRAIL OF THE ASSASSINS
BY JIM GARRISON

Jim Garrison was District Attorney of New Orleans at the time of the Kennedy assassination. His book *On the Trail of the Assassins* was published in 1988, and it describes first hand his efforts to bring Kennedy's killers to justice. The book served as the basis for the Oliver Stone film *JFK*.

His story opens on the day of the assassination. Like most Americans Garrison was stunned to learn of JFK's sudden demise, and he remained glued to the TV set of a French Quarter restaurant as events unfolded. By midafternoon it was announced that Dallas police had surrounded and apprehended the prime suspect in a movie theater several miles from the assassination site. His name was Lee Harvey Oswald.

Garrison soon became aware of another significant event that was

94

unfolding that afternoon several blocks away in the office of private detective Guy Banister. Banister was the former FBI special agent in charge of the Bureau's Chicago office. He had previously served as deputy superintendent of the New Orleans Police Department, and had gained a reputation as a solid proponent of law and order. Garrison knew Banister well, having lunched with him on several occasions, swapping stories about their earlier careers in the FBI.

The afternoon of the assassination Banister had been drinking heavily in a French Quarter bar with office associate Jack Martin. Upon returning to the office, Martin reminded Banister of the strange events he had witnessed the previous summer, including the presence of Lee Harvey Oswald in the office, whereupon Banister unholstered his .357 Magnum and used it to smash in Martin's skull, sending him to the hospital. The event was recorded in New Orleans Police Department report K-12634-63.

Soon after the beating Martin confided to a friend that David Ferrie, another Banister associate and well known adventurer and pilot, had hastily left New Orleans for Texas an hour after the assassination, ostensibly to provide "getaway" services for the assassins. This information soon reaches Garrison, who initiates an investigation into Ferrie. Garrison had previously met Ferrie in a chance encounter on the streets of New Orleans, noting his bizarre appearance,* and was well aware of Ferrie's reputation for anti-Castro and anti-Communist activities.

Garrison soon learns that Oswald spent three months of the previous summer in New Orleans and decides to extend his investigation to include Oswald's activities during that time. Looking into Oswald's conduct that summer, investigators soon discover that Oswald had been seen with Ferrie.

Garrison's detectives visit Ferrie's apartment and find a cache of military equipment and a large map of Cuba on the wall. Ferrie is soon located, and he explains that his trip to Texas was to go ice skating in Houston. Investigators learn that Ferrie did indeed visit an ice skating rink in Houston, but instead of ice skating, he spent his time on a pay phone, making and receiving calls. Ferrie continued on to Galveston, and was there when Jack Ruby called Galveston the night before he shot and killed Lee Harvey Oswald.

Garrison orders Ferrie to be taken into custody for questioning by the

---

* Ferrie suffered from alopecia areata, a disease that causes the loss of all body hair, and as a result wore a wig and painted on his eyebrows.

FBI, who quickly arrange for his release. As a result Garrison concludes that the FBI had found no connection between Ferrie and the assassination. Having delivered his suspicions to the FBI, Garrison felt confident that the matter would be fully investigated, and he turned his attention back to the more mundane matters of crime in New Orleans.*

Three years pass and Garrison has a chance conversation with Russell Long, the U.S. senator from Louisiana. Long states that the members of the Warren Commission "were dead wrong", and that "There's no way in the world that one man could have shot up Jack Kennedy that way." The conversation rekindles Garrison's interest in the assassination, and he orders a full 26 volume set of the Warren Commission's investigation and findings.

While waiting for the volumes to arrive, he researches the Commission's origins and composition. Five days after the assassination Representative Charles Goodell proposed a joint Congressional Committee to examine the assassination, but before congress could act, newly inaugurated President Lyndon Johnson announced that he had already created an investigative commission.** Garrison notes that the Commission's composition was top-heavy with individuals from the intelligence community: Alan Dulles was a former Director of the CIA who had been fired by Kennedy, John McCloy was a former Assistant Secretary for the Department of War, and Representative Gerald Ford was, according to *Newsweek* magazine, "the CIA's best friend in Congress".

Garrison carefully studies the Commission's findings and notes the same glaring discrepancies between witness testimony and the Commission's conclusions that were observed by Mark Lane. He is intrigued by the fact that numerous witnesses and police heard shots from the grassy knoll, but were turned away by individuals flashing Secret Service credentials when they attempted to access the railroad yard and parking lot behind the knoll. The Secret Service denied that any of their agents were there.

---

* Garrison notes that when the House Select Committee on Assassinations concluded that President Kennedy was probably assassinated "as the result of a conspiracy", it found an apparent association between David Ferrie and Lee Harvey Oswald in New Orleans.

** In a recorded telephone conversation with FBI director J. Edgar Hoover, Johnson discussed the formation of a commission with the express purpose of thwarting a congressional investigation (Chapter 1).

Garrison soon returns to Oswald's activities during the summer of 1963, and focuses on the 544 Camp Street address that was hand stamped on leaflets that Oswald handed out for the "Fair Play for Cuba Committee". Guy Banister died in 1964, but Garrison determines that 544 Camp Street was near the former location of "Guy Banister Associates, Inc., Investigators" at 531 Lafayette Street, and, in fact, both entrances led to the same place – Guy Banister's office.

Garrison knew that Banister had previously hired and directed individuals to pose as sympathetic *agents provocateurs* to penetrate leftist organizations, and that as head of the Anti-Communist League of the Caribbean, he could easily have done the same with Oswald. His suspicions were only heightened by the fact that Oswald routinely visited unemployment offices to recruit paid leafleteers to assist him, despite lacking the financial resources to do so.

While visiting 544 Camp Street, Garrison notes that several federal intelligence agencies are located in the vicinity of Banister's former office. The New Orleans division of the Secret Service is housed in the U.S. Post Office building directly across the street, as is the Office of Naval Intelligence, to which Banister once belonged. The CIA is located just a few blocks away in a building known as the Masonic Temple, as was the FBI in the early 1960s. He wonders if it was just a coincidence that Banister's office and Oswald's activities were both located in the heart of the federal intelligence apparatus in New Orleans.

Garrison interviews Jack Martin and confirms that both David Ferrie and Lee Harvey Oswald were frequent visitors to Banister's office, and that all three were substantially involved in efforts to accumulate and deliver military hardware to anti-Castro Cubans. He locates and interviews Banister's widow, who tells him that federal agents arrived at Banister's office within hours of his death to take away several locked filing cabinets, and that afterward the state police came and departed with the index cards to Banister's files. Garrison dispatches an investigator to visit the Louisiana State Police headquarters in Baton Rouge, and the remains of the index cards are located. They confirm the true nature of Guy Banister's operation: American Central Intelligence Agency, 20-10; Fair Play for Cuba Committee, 23-7; International Trade Mart, 23-14; Ammunition and Arms, 32-1.

The trail of armaments leads to former CIA employee Gordon Novel and his efforts to remove land mines and grenades stored in a Schlumberger Corporation bunker in Houma, Louisiana.* The seized armaments were divided equally between David Ferrie's apartment and Guy Banister's office for temporary storage and eventual transport.

Garrison obtains a summary of the Secret Service report for the investigation of 544 Camp Street indicating that "no one at that address had ever recalled seeing Lee Harvey Oswald" and that "nothing of consequence had been found at that address." Garrison notes that 544 Camp Street is fifty feet from the front entrance to the New Orleans division of the Secret Service, and had investigators climbed the stairs at 544 Camp Street they would have found themselves at Guy Banister's office, whose secretary, Delphine Roberts, could have told them that "Banister had engaged in closed-door meetings with Oswald and that he had arranged for a third-floor room for Oswald's use."

Soon Garrison focuses on Commission testimony concerning Oswald's background, and particularly the fact that Oswald's service record shows that he had taken a Russian examination at the El Toro Marine Base in California. Knowledge of Russian is not a standard part of service training and Garrison concludes that Oswald was being prepared for intelligence work. He continues to review Oswald's assignment at El Toro from November 1958 to September 1959, and determines that with one exception, no one remembered Oswald as espousing Socialist, Marxist, Communist, anti-American, or anti-Capitalist ideals. That one exception was Kerry Thornley, an Oswald look-alike who Garrison later suspects of masquerading as Oswald to promote the image of Oswald as a fanatical Communist.

Oswald was discharged from the Marines in September 1959, and the following month he defected to the Soviet Union.** He was sent to Minsk, where he met and married Marina Prusakova, niece of a lieutenant colonel

---

* Schlumberger is a large French-owned geological services corporation known to have supported the French Secret Army Organization, which attempted to assassinate French President Charles de Gaulle several times in the 1950s and 60s.

** Garrison notes that in testimony before the House Select Committee on Assassinations, former CIA finance officer James A. Wilcott reported that Oswald had been recruited from the military by the CIA "with the express purpose of a double agent assignment in the USSR".

in the KGB. He returned to the United States in June 1962, without any of the questions, interference, or obstruction one might generally expect to confront a former defector to the Soviet Union, and in fact was met in New York by Spas T. Raikin, secretary general of the American Friends of the Anti-Bolshevik Nations, Inc. According to the Warren Commission, Raikin had been asked by the State Department to render any required aid to the Oswalds.

After returning to the United States Oswald becomes acquainted with George de Mohrenschildt, a prominent member of the White Russian community in Dallas.* De Mohrenschildt worked for French intelligence during World War II. He was highly educated, spoke several languages fluently, and is thought to have had substantial connections to the CIA. Among de Mohrenshildt's close friends was Jean de Menil, president of Schlumberger. De Mohrenschildt was found shotgunned to death in March 1977 after arranging to meet with an investigator for the House Select Committee on Assassinations. He is known to have viewed Oswald as an innocent scapegoat.

Shortly after meeting de Mohrenschildt, Oswald began employment at Jagger-Stovall-Chiles doing high security work for Pentagon related top-secret U-2 missions. Garrison observes that it is highly unlikely that an ardent Communist could have obtained the security clearance necessary to perform this type of work.

De Mohrenschildt introduces Oswald to Ruth Paine, whose family was well connected to federal security organizations: her husband did highly classified work for a major Department of Defense contractor, her father had worked for the Agency for International Development, long regarded as a CIA front organization, and her brother-in-law worked for the same agency in Washington.

Paine speaks fluent Russian, and she soon becomes friends with Oswald's wife, Marina. After their stay in New Orleans during the summer of 1963, Paine drives Marina Oswald and her daughter back to Dallas, and provides them with a place to live in her house. Lee Oswald soon follows, and Paine arranges for him to obtain a job at the Texas School Book Depository in

* The term "White Russian" refers to individuals and groups who were opposed to the 1917 Bolshevik takeover of the Soviet Union, many of whom eventually fled to other nations.

October 1963.

In the course of his investigation, Garrison attempts to obtain the tax records of both Ruth and Michael Paine, but he is told that they have been classified as secret. He notes that numerous Commission documents related to Ruth and Michael Paine, and their relatives, have been classified as secret on the grounds of national security.

According to the Warren Commission Report, prior to starting his job at the Texas School Book Depository Oswald traveled to Mexico City to visit the Soviet and Cuban embassies. After the report was issued, the CIA produced surveillance photos and audio tapes made at those embassies during that time, allegedly showing Oswald. It was easily determined, however, that the person in the photos and the voice on the tapes did not resemble Oswald.

Garrison recounts an incident in early November 1963 in which an individual identifying himself as Lee Oswald took a car out on a test drive, drove memorably like a maniac, and then made loud complaints that included references of going "back to Russia" and that he would soon be coming into some money. Garrison believes that Kerry Thornley may have been impersonating Oswald to lay the groundwork for the lone-gunman-crazed-Communist persona into which Oswald would soon be thrust. He notes the parallels between Oswald's movements and Thornley's travel to New Orleans, Dallas, and Mexico.

In early 1968 Garrison locates Thornley in Tampa and subpoenas him to testify before a Grand Jury in New Orleans. Thornley admits to having met Guy Banister and David Ferrie in New Orleans. While living in New Orleans in 1963 he rented an apartment from John Spencer, a friend of Clay Shaw, who would soon become a pivotal figure in Garrison's investigation. Thornley left New Orleans for Washington soon after the assassination, where he was found to have been living beyond his means in an expensive first-class apartment. Thornley eventually becomes friends with John Roselli, who was subsequently murdered after his Senate testimony on CIA assassination practices.

Garrison then examines the Warren Commission testimony of New Orleans lawyer Dean Andrews, who told the Commission that he had received a call shortly after the assassination to represent Lee Harvey Oswald. The caller was Clay Bertrand, who had previously provided Andrews with legal work. Garrison soon learns that Clay Bertrand is an alias used by Clay Shaw, a prominent member of New Orleans society who was the director of the International Trade Mart.

Clay Shaw had been employed by the CIA in their efforts to provide financial support to the paramilitary right in Europe with the goal of suppressing Communism.

He was a director of the Centro Mondiale Commerciale (World Trade Center), formed initially in Montreal, then moved to Rome in 1961, as well as Permindex, a related company created in Switzerland by the Centro Mondiale. The Centro Mondiale and Permindex were unmasked and expelled from Europe in 1962, settling in Johannesburg, South Africa. Both are thought to have been creations of the CIA.

In 1967 the Canadian newspaper *Le Devoir* published an article about the Centro Mondiale Commerciale and one of its directors, Ferenc Nagy, who had substantial links to the CIA and anti-Castro Cubans living in Miami. Nagy eventually moved to the U.S., settling in Dallas.

Le Devoir went on to discuss the role of Major Louis Mortimer Bloomfield, an American living in Montreal, who had been an agent for the Office of Strategic Services (OSS), predecessor of the CIA. The paper stated that Bloomfield had been involved in espionage for the U.S. in earlier years, and was a major shareholder in the Centro Mondiale and Permindex.

The Italian newspaper *Paesa Sera* stated that the "Center was a creature of the CIA…set up as a cover for the transfer of CIA…funds in Italy for illegal political-espionage activities. It still remains to clear up the presence on the administrative Board of the Center of Clay Shaw and ex-Major (of the OSS) Bloomfield." Permindex was also accused of financing the French Secret Army Organization's (OAS) attempts to assassinate French President Charles de Gaulle.

Uncovering a connection between Clay Shaw and Lee Harvey Oswald moves Garrison's investigation in a new direction, but he bemoans the fact that he became aware of the connection between Shaw, Permindex, the Centro Mondiale, and the CIA too late to be of help in his investigation.

Turning back to the events in Dealey Plaza, Garrison notes the confusion that arose out of Officer Seymour Weitzman's initial identification of the murder weapon as a 7.65 caliber German Mauser, as opposed to the Italian made Mannlicher-Carcano that was eventually tied to Oswald. Weitzman operated a sporting goods store and was a recognized authority on weapons. The misidentification suggests the possibility that two weapons were found on the sixth floor.

Garrison's suspicions are heightened when he learns that the original parade route was changed the morning of the assassination to pass directly under the sixth floor window, and that the mayor of Dallas, Earle Cabell, was the brother of General Charles Cabell, former Deputy Director of the CIA who was fired by Kennedy.

The Warren Commission version of the altered parade route was shown as a copy of the front page of the *Dallas Morning News* that had the parade route replaced by a solid gray square. At that point Garrison begins to view the assassination as a *coup d'etat*.

The investigation progresses and Garrison uncovers interlocking connections between David Ferrie, Clay Shaw, Lee Harvey Oswald, and Jack Ruby. He learns of a flight to Montreal piloted by David Ferrie. The trip included Clay Shaw and Jules Ricco Kimble, an individual associated with extreme right groups such as the Ku Klux Klan. Upon landing in Montreal, Shaw disappears and returns the next day with a man of "Mexican or Cuban" appearance for transport back to the U.S.. Garrison notes that Major Louis Mortimer Bloomfield resided in Montreal at the time of the trip.

Garrison describes an attempt by Ferrie and Shaw to recruit Edward Whalen, a professional criminal, to kill him in order to stop his investigation. Whalen describes a meeting that included Ferrie, Shaw, and, for a period of time, attorney Dean Andrews. After Andrews had left, Ferrie, using Shaw's Bertrand alias, describes how Shaw had done a lot for Oswald, and it was only because Oswald "had fouled up" that he had to be killed. Ferrie states that Oswald was an agent of the CIA. Garrison believes that Andrews tipped off Ferrie and Shaw as to his ongoing investigation of the assassination.

As news of the investigation seeps out of his office, Garrison becomes the target of media harassment. He is visited by John Miller, a self-described oil man from Denver, who promises him a federal judgeship if he abandons the investigation. Garrison's staff note the Annapolis ring that Miller was wearing.

Garrison and his staff debate calling Ferrie before a Grand Jury. Ferrie contacts Garrison's office complaining about media harassment, and remarks to one of Garrison's investigators that "I'm a dead man now". Garrison's office provides him with alternate accommodations, but he soon turns up dead in his apartment, along with two suicide notes and an empty bottle of Proloid. The coroner rules that he died of natural causes.

Shaw is soon arrested for conspiracy to murder the President, and his apartment is searched. At his booking he is asked if he used any aliases, and he replies "Clay Bertrand", confirming to Garrison that Shaw is the individual who contacted Dean Andrews to represent Oswald. His address book reads like a Who's Who of European royalty, but one item in particular interests Garrison: LEE ODOM, P.O. Box 19106, Dallas, Texas. The same address had appeared in Oswald's address book.

Shaw's attorneys produce one Lee Odom from Irving, a suburb of Dallas, who states that the box number had been used by a barbecue company with which he had once been associated. He explains that he had met Clay Shaw to promote a bullfight in New Orleans. Garrison is puzzled by the fact that P.O. Box 19106 was issued after 1963, the year in which Oswald died, yet was contained in Oswald's address book.

Oswald's address book also contained the name and unlisted phone number of FBI Agent James Hosty, both of which were excluded in the Warren Commission's listing of the book's contents. Garrison considers the possibility that Oswald was an FBI confidential informant, and that this was the source of Waggoner Carr's allegations that Oswald had been working for the FBI. Oswald visited the Dallas FBI office shortly before the assassination and left a note for Hosty. After the assassination Hosty was ordered to burn the note by Gordon Shanklin, Special Agent in Charge of the Dallas Office.

The search of Shaw's apartment turns up additional items: five blood-encrusted whips, lengths of chain, and a black hood with matching cape. Investigators note two large hooks screwed into Shaw's bedroom ceiling.

Shaw's arrest precipitates a fierce counterattack by the federal government and national media. Garrison is denounced by Attorney General Ramsey Clark, as well as the Chief Justice of the Supreme Court, Earl Warren. Clark announced that Shaw had been investigated by the FBI and cleared of any involvement with the assassination. Garrison wonders why Shaw was investigated in the first place, if he had nothing to do with the assassination. Shortly afterward, the Justice Department announced that it was aware that Clay Bertrand and Clay Shaw were the same individual and that Bertrand had been investigated.

With Ferrie dead, Garrison is forced to rely on other witnesses to move the case forward. Perry Russo, a 25 year old Equitable insurance salesman, becomes his most important witness. Russo was a longtime friend of

David Ferrie, and was present at a meeting with Ferrie and Shaw where the assassination of Kennedy was openly discussed. Also at the meeting was an individual introduced as "Leon" Oswald. Russo could not confirm that the Leon Oswald at the meeting was the same person he saw on television, accused of the assassination.

In the spring of 1967 a special NBC investigative team arrives in New Orleans. The team is headed by Walter Sheridan, who frequently makes references to his prior service in the Office of Naval Intelligence. Garrison receives a memo from Marlene Mancuso, the former wife of Gordon Novel, the CIA linked operative who participated in the removal of land mines and grenades stored in the Schlumberger bunker in Houma, Louisiana. Garrison was trying to extradite Novel from Ohio back to Louisiana. Mancuso warns Garrison that NBC is actively looking for information to discredit his investigation.

According to Perry Russo, Walter Sheridan told him that the president of NBC had contacted senior management at his employer, Equitable Insurance, and Sheridan went on to make thinly veiled threats about his continued employment with Equitable. Sheridan offered to set him up in California and protect his job if Russo would cease cooperation with Garrison's probe. Sheridan also told Russo that NBC had flown Gordon Novel to Virginia, and that Garrison would never get him back to Louisiana.

As the investigation progresses, Garrison begins to see overwhelming CIA involvement in Oswald's pre-assassination activities, including his contacts with Banister, Shaw, and Ferrie. While awaiting possible extradition back to Louisiana, Gordon Novel gives interviews and press conferences in Ohio in which he declares that the removal of armaments from the Schlumberger bunker in Houma had been at the direction of the CIA, and that everyone present, including David Ferrie, had been working for the CIA.

Garrison's attempt to extradite Novel is blocked, as is his attempt to extradite Sandra Moffett, Perry Russo's girlfriend, who was present at the party that preceded Russo's discussions with Shaw, Ferrie, and "Leon" Oswald concerning the assassination of the President.

Garrison describes meeting Richard Case Nagell, a former federal intelligence agent, who told him that he had been assigned to work with Oswald, and that by September 1963 he had detected that an "exceedingly large operation pointing to the assassination of President Kennedy was under way". He contacted J. Edgar Hoover via registered mail to warn him of the plot, only to be ignored.

Garrison documents other tactics intended to derail his investigation. His office was infiltrated by former CIA agent Bill Boxley, who Garrison believes provided copies of all of his files to the federal government. Garrison describes Boxley's attempt to set him up for a homosexual sting arrest in the men's room of the Los Angeles airport.

Shaw is eventually brought to trial for conspiracy to murder President Kennedy. At that point Garrison had been deprived of the testimony of three of his most important witnesses – David Ferrie, Gordon Novel, and Sandra Moffett – and he was forced to use testimony from less credible individuals to connect Shaw to Ferrie and Oswald.

The trial soon focuses on the physical evidence of a conspiracy to murder the President, including the Zapruder film showing Kennedy's head snapping back and to the left from a shot that could only have come from in front.*

In response, the defense calls one of the three military pathologists who conducted Kennedy's autopsy, Lieutenant Colonel Pierre Finck.** Finck's testimony supports the Warren Commission's conclusion that Kennedy was struck by two bullets fired from behind, but when challenged by prosecutors as to why the wounds of the neck were not probed and dissected, he testifies that the pathologists were ordered not to do so.

Clay Shaw takes the stand and testifies that he had never known David Ferrie or Lee Harvey Oswald, had never used the alias Clay Bertrand, and had never called Dean Andrews. Garrison is surprised that Shaw denied knowing Ferrie, because the numerous witnesses linking the two would invite a future perjury prosecution.

Shaw is acquitted. Interviews of the jurors afterwards established that the jury believed that Kennedy was killed as the result of a conspiracy, but

---

* Garrison notes that the FBI originally supplied the Warren Commission with a copy of the Zapruder film that had frames 314 and 315 reversed, showing the president's head moving forward, indicating a shot from the rear. J. Edgar Hoover attributed the reversal to an "inadvertent" printing error.

** Finck also participated in the autopsy of Robert Kennedy after his assassination on June 4, 1968.

could not find any motive for Shaw to have participated in such a conspiracy.

Garrison is incensed that Shaw "had taken the witness stand and, in his grand and courtly manner, made a mockery of the law against lying under oath". He files perjury charges against Shaw for having testified that he had never met David Ferrie. The United States District Court takes the unusual step of enjoining Garrison from prosecuting Shaw, effectively ending the case.

Clay Shaw would be dead within a few years, expiring under mysterious circumstances. Shaw's neighbor saw a body being carried into Shaw's house on a stretcher covered by a sheet. The New Orleans coroner was notified and soon learns that Shaw's body had been quickly buried in nearby Kentwood. Sensing the possibility of foul play, the coroner attempts to exhume the body for examination, but media pressure puts an end to the inquiry.

The federal government soon prosecutes Garrison for allegedly taking protection money from pinball game operators. The judge for the trial is Herbert Christenberry, the same judge who signed the order prohibiting Garrison from prosecuting Shaw for perjury. The government's case collapses when its star witness is shown to have given an interview in which he indicates that the federal government is forcing him to lie on their behalf, and that their case against Garrison is a fraud. Audio tapes against Garrison are also shown to have been doctored. Garrison is acquitted.

After the Shaw trial, Garrison learns that the CIA had more than a passing interest in the outcome. In an article published in 1975, Victor Marchetti, who, at the time, had been a high-ranking staff employee at CIA Headquarters, revealed that CIA Director Richard Helms would inquire at staff meetings if Shaw's team was getting "all the help they need", and that Shaw and Ferrie had both worked for the CIA.

HIGH TREASON
BY ROBERT GRODEN AND HARRISON LIVINGSTONE

High Treason: The Assassination of President John F. Kennedy - What Really Happened was published in 1989 by Robert Groden and Harrison Livingstone. Groden had worked as a Staff Photographic Consultant for the House Select Committee on Assassinations, and was intimately familiar with the photographic aspects of the assassination. He was the driving force behind the presentation of the Zapruder film to the American public for the first time on Geraldo Rivera's television variety show in 1975, and he also worked as a consultant on the Oliver Stone film *JFK*.

Harrison Livingstone is a prominent Kennedy assassination researcher who wrote a follow-up work entitled *High Treason 2*, amplifying many of the themes and ideas that appeared in the original.

Groden and Livingstone's book is an encyclopedic catalog of the various alleged misdeeds and frauds perpetrated by federal officials and the Warren Commission in the wake of Kennedy's death.

In their scenario, Groden and Livingstone envision a fusillade of shots fired at the President:

1. The first shot occurs around Zapruder Frame 155 and misses the President, causing the film to blur from Zapruder's reaction to the sound.

2. The next shot is from the front and hits the President in the throat, causing him to clutch at his throat.

3. The next shot hits the President in the back six inches below the shoulder, just to the right of his spinal column.

4. The next shot hits Governor Connally in the back, just under the right armpit.

5. A bullet then strikes the inside chrome above the windshield of the President's limousine, followed by another that hits the sidewalk alongside the limousine.

6. The President is then struck in the head twice, with shots from the front and back arriving nearly simultaneously at Zapruder Frames 312 and 313, possibly merging into the sound of a single shot.

7. Six-tenths of a second later Governor Connally is shot in the wrist, and then the bullet passes into his thigh.

8. The final bullet hits bystander James Tague in the cheek after ricocheting off the sidewalk near where Elm Street goes under the railroad underpass.*

---

* The paperback version of *High Treason*, however, opens with a best fit

In a chapter entitled "Strange Deaths" Groden and Livingstone enumerate the many mysterious deaths related to the Kennedy assassination, including:

1. Guy Banister: former head of the Chicago FBI office with substantial CIA connections; he is thought to have directed Oswald's activities in New Orleans during the summer of 1963; died in 1964.

2. Albert Guy Bogard: allegedly took Oswald on a test drive at a Lincoln-Mercury dealership; stated that Oswald told him that he might have to "go back to Russia" and would soon be coming into "a lot of money"; found dead in 1966 with a hose connected to the exhaust pipe of his car.*

3. Hale Boggs: one of seven Commissioners on the Warren Commission; publicly expressed doubts about the single bullet theory promoted by Arlen Specter and Gerald Ford; publicly criticized the FBI and accused J. Edgar Hoover of engaging in Gestapo tactics; disappeared without a trace in a plane crash over Alaska.

4. Lee Bowers, Jr.: viewed the assassination from a railroad tower overlooking the parking lot behind the grassy knoll and provided significant eyewitness testimony to events in the parking lot before and during the assassination; died in a single car crash in 1966.

5. Karen Bennett Carlin (also known as Teresa Norton and Little Lynn): stripper who worked for Jack Ruby; shot to death in August

---

version of the House Select Committee acoustic data: Shot #1 from behind, Shot #2 from behind, Shot #3 from the right front, Shot #4 from behind.

* Groden and Livingstone point out another connection to the Lincoln-Mercury dealership where Albert Guy Bogard worked. An individual named Jack Lawrence worked there for one month before the assassination. He borrowed a car from the dealership the night before the assassination and reported for work thirty minutes afterward in an unkempt, muddied, and nauseous condition. Dealership employees retrieved the car from the parking lot behind the Grassy Knoll and called the police, who arrested Lawrence and held him for a day. He was frequently seen in Jack Ruby's Carousel strip club and is thought to have been a close friend of Ruby's roommate George Senator. He was also known to be an expert marksman.

1964 in Houston.

6. Rose Cherami: Ruby employee who was thrown from a moving car by two Ruby associates before the assassination; at the hospital she foretold of the assassination, and later stated that Oswald and Ruby were "bedmates"; died in a hit and run accident in 1965.

7. Bill Chesher: thought to have information linking Ruby and Oswald; died of a heart attack in March 1964.

8. Dr. Nicholas Chetta: Coroner of New Orleans at the time of Jim Garrison's investigation of Clay Shaw; performed autopsies on several dead witnesses connected to Garrison's investigation, including David Ferrie; died of a heart attack in May 1968.

9. George de Mohrenschildt: Russian friend of the Oswalds who had substantial CIA and international contacts; he was found shotgunned to death after being contacted by an investigator from the House Select Committee on Assassinations; his death was ruled a suicide.

10. Aladio del Valle: close friend of David Ferrie who was sought by Jim Garrison as a witness; died at the same time as David Ferrie as the result of having his skull split open with a machete and being shot in the heart.

11. David Ferrie: key witness in Jim Garrison's investigation of Clay Shaw; Ferrie had substantial connections to Oswald, Shaw and the CIA, as well as New Orleans Mafia godfather Carlos Marcello; died of a brain hemorrhage in February 1967.

12. Maurice Brooks Gatlin, Sr.: CIA associate of Guy Banister; fell from a hotel window in Panama in 1964.

13. Sam Giancana: Mafia figure who was involved in CIA plots against Castro; shot in his basement before he could testify before the House Select Committee on Assassinations; his daughter thought that he was "killed by the same people who killed Kennedy".

14. Thomas Hale Howard: Ruby's lawyer; he was at Ruby's apartment the night after Ruby shot Oswald; died of a heart attack.

15. Bill Hunter: newspaper writer who was at Ruby's apartment the night after Ruby shot Oswald; shot to death in a police station in Long Beach, California in April 1964.

16. Clyde Johnson: knew of a personal relationship between Oswald, Ruby, Shaw and Ferrie; beaten the day before he was to testify at Clay Shaw's trial and died of a shotgun wound shortly afterwards.

17. Regis Kennedy: FBI agent; died in 1978 after talking to the House Select Committee on Assassinations.

18. Dorothy Kilgallen: prominent media personality and columnist who interviewed Jack Ruby and claimed that she would break the assassination "wide open"; died in November 1965 of a drug overdose that was ruled a suicide.

19. Henry Killam: husband of Wanda Joyce Killam, who knew Ruby since 1947 and worked for him from July 1963 through November 1963; died from having his throat slit in March 1964, after having told his brother that he was "a dead man".

20. Jim Koethe: was at Ruby's apartment the night after Ruby shot Oswald; assaulted and killed in his Dallas apartment in September 1964.

21. Betty Mooney MacDonald (also known as Nancy Jane Mooney): stripper who worked for Jack Ruby; she provided an alibi for Darrell Wayne Garner, who was accused of shooting assassination witness Warren Reynolds; she was also at a private party with the Oswalds and the de Mohrenschildts; arrested in February 1964 and found hanging in her jail cell.

22. Robert Perrin: known gun-runner and husband of Nancy Perrin Rich, who testified that Jack Ruby was involved in Cuban arms smuggling; dead of arsenic poisoning.

23. Lieutenant Commander William Bruce Pitzer: head of the Bethesda Naval Hospital audio-visual unit at the time of the assassination; reportedly took photographs of the autopsy, although his name does not appear on the official FBI log of those in attendance; he was found shot to death in his office at Bethesda Naval Hospital in October 1966; the death was ruled a suicide.*

24. Carlos Prio: former President of Cuba; shot to death before the House Select Committee on Assassinations could speak with him.

25. Earlene Roberts: housekeeper at Oswald's rooming house; testified that shortly after the assassination a police car stopped in front of the house and honked its horn twice while Oswald was inside; she also stated that an "Officer Alexander", thought to have been prominent right wing Assistant District Attorney Bill Alexander, a known associate of Jack Ruby, was sometimes at the house; she died of heart failure in January 1966.

26. Johnny Roselli: Mafia figure who was involved in CIA plots against Castro; connected to Sam Giancana through the Chicago underworld; he hinted that he knew who killed Kennedy; murdered after providing Senate testimony.

---

* The History Channel has presented testimony from Dennis David, a former hospital colleague of Pitzer's, stating that Pitzer showed him photographs from the autopsy that display a small wound in the President's right temple and a huge gaping hole in the back of his head. The History Channel presented further testimony from Daniel Marvin, a highly decorated Green Beret who attended specialist guerrilla training at Fort Bragg, North Carolina. Part of his training involved top secret instruction in assassination and terrorism conducted in a separate, heavily guarded facility that included a model of Dealey Plaza to illustrate how an assassination is organized and constructed to throw blame on one individual and then covered up afterward. He was told that Oswald was not involved in the assassination. Fifteen months later he and another individual, Captain David H. Vanek, were taken to meet with an official from the CIA. Marvin was asked individually if he would volunteer to assassinate an American naval officer, who he presumed was located outside the United States. He tentatively agreed and was given the name of William Bruce Pitzer, but ultimately declined the assignment upon learning that Pitzer was located in the U.S.. He never saw Vanek again, and his subsequent attempt to locate Vanek was met with an official denial that Vanek ever existed, despite Marvin having official published orders to the contrary. [2]

27. Clay Shaw: central figure in Jim Garrison's investigation into Oswald's activities the summer before the assassination; he had substantial connections to the CIA; died mysteriously in 1974, reportedly of lung cancer.

28. Dr. Mary Sherman: associate of David Ferrie; shot in bed and set on fire.

29. Mrs. Earl T. Smith: close friend and confidante of Dorothy Kilgallen; died of indeterminate causes two days after Kilgallen died.

30. William Sullivan: number three man at the FBI under J. Edgar Hoover; he wrote a book entitled *The Bureau* that was critical of Hoover; he was shot to death in a hunting accident in 1977 before he could speak to the House Select Committee on Assassinations.

31. Gary Underhill: former CIA agent who fled Washington after the assassination; he told friends that the CIA was involved in the assassination; he was shot in the left side of his head and his death was ruled a suicide, although he was right-handed.

32. Deputy Sheriff Buddy Walthers: found a bullet in the grass near Elm Street, and turned it over to an individual representing himself to be an FBI agent; shot through the heart in a police shootout in 1969.

33. Hugh Ward: Guy Banister's partner; died in a plane crash in Mexico in 1964, along with the mayor of New Orleans.

34. William Whaley: cab driver who drove Oswald away from the assassination site; died in a car accident while on duty in December 1965, the first Dallas cab driver fatality since 1937.

High Treason places a great deal of emphasis on the government-produced autopsy photographs and X-rays as a prime example of the fraudulent nature of the investigation. Groden and Livingstone maintain that the Warren Commission never examined the autopsy photographs and X-rays due to political pressure, but clearly if the Commission had decided to publish these transparently fabricated materials, it would have had the impossible task of displaying them alongside the medical testimony from

Parkland Hospital and the Bethesda autopsy records, which are completely contradictory.

A common theme throughout *High Treason* is the presence of a "Secret Team" in government, a concept described by Colonel Fletcher Prouty in a book of the same name. Colonel Prouty served as liaison between the Pentagon and the CIA, and was in a position to have first hand knowledge of the dark machinations of government. According to Prouty, the Secret Team is a group of highly influential men from industry, banking, military and legal circles who are in a position to manipulate government policy by controlling the activities of key individuals within government. The Secret Team began to exert its influence around 1959, and played a key role in arranging Kennedy's murder and its subsequent cover-up. Groden and Livingstone believe that Richard Nixon was a member of the Secret Team.

Groden and Livingstone discuss the "Three Tramps" and their importance to understanding the assassination. Immediately after the assassination the police focused a great deal of attention on the parking lot and railroad yard behind the grassy knoll. Eventually three vagabonds were located in a rail car about to leave the yard, and they were paraded into police headquarters. Many of the news photographers took their photos. They were never heard from again and there is no police record of their presence at headquarters.

Photographs of the tramps show individuals who are wearing clean clothing in good repair, well maintained shoes, and who display a high level of personal grooming, suggesting that they may not have been the itinerant travelers they represented themselves to be.

A photograph of the tramps is shown in Figure 5-7. Groden and Livingstone note that the older tramp appears to be E. Howard Hunt, a CIA operative and prominent figure in the Watergate scandal. The taller tramp is thought to resemble Frank Sturgis, another CIA operative and participant in the Watergate break-in.*

---

* More recent interpretations of the "Three Tramps" photos suggest that they were Chauncey Holt, Charles Rogers, and Charles Harrelson. Holt was a career criminal who did work for the Mafia's Meyer Lansky and William Harvey of the CIA. Charles Rogers, known to Holt as Richard Montoya, was a convicted killer thought to have dismembered and chopped up the bodies of his parents. Charles Harrelson was convicted of killing a federal judge and is known to have bragged about killing President Kennedy. [3]

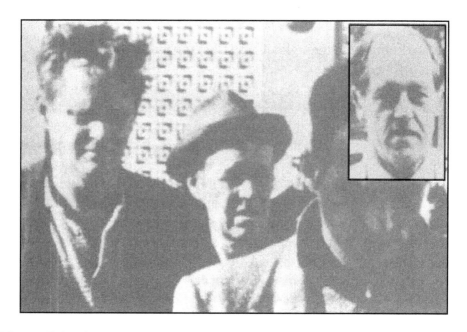

Figure 5-7. Photograph of the Three Tramps. Inset, upper right, photograph of E. Howard Hunt.

E. Howard Hunt was a close friend of Warren Commissioner Allen Dulles, head of the CIA until he was forced to resign by President Kennedy in 1961 over the Bay of Pigs debacle. Hunt is thought to have ghost-written Dulles' book *The Craft of Intelligence.*

Groden and Livingstone go on to discuss the connection between the Kennedy assassination and the Watergate scandal, events that on the surface appear to have nothing in common. The Watergate scandal began the evening of June 17, 1972, when five burglars were arrested for breaking into the Democratic Party's national headquarters in the Watergate complex of apartments and offices in Washington.

After the arrests President Nixon authorized payments of "hush money" in an attempt to quiet the accused, but a wide ranging campaign of political espionage, sabotage, and dirty tricks emanating from the White House was soon uncovered, eventually leading to the resignation of President Nixon and sending others to jail.

E. Howard Hunt was accused of masterminding the burglary, and served

33 months in prison for burglary, conspiracy, and wiretapping. The presence of Hunt in Dealey Plaza directly connects Watergate and the Kennedy assassination.*

Testimony from Marita Lorenz to the House Select Committee on Assassinations places Watergate burglar Frank Sturgis at the center of events leading up to the assassination. In 1959 Lorenz was living with Fidel Castro when she was recruited by Sturgis to work for the CIA. Lorenz testified that a few days before the assassination, she drove with Sturgis from Miami to Dallas in a two car caravan laden with weapons.

Groden and Livingstone also note a curious connection between Richard Nixon and Jack Ruby that emerged in 1947 from the House Committee on Un-American Activities, of which Nixon was a member. Nixon intervened on behalf of a Chicago gangster who was to testify before the committee. An FBI staff assistant wrote: "It is my sworn statement that one Jack Rubenstein of Chicago, noted as a potential witness for hearings of the House Committee on Un-American Activities, is performing functions for the staff of Congressman Richard Nixon, Republican of California. It is requested Rubenstein not be called for open testimony in the aforementioned hearings."

At the time, Ruby was a Chicago gangster known as Jack Rubenstein. He legally changed his name to Jack Ruby after moving to Dallas in 1947.

Many date the beginning of the Kennedy assassination plot to the rise of Fidel Castro and his installation of Communism in Cuba. Prior to Castro's arrival the Mafia made millions of dollars every day through their casinos, prostitution, and other enterprises in Havana. Havana was a paradise playground just 90 miles from U.S. shores where they could escape the scrutiny and reach of American justice and do as they pleased. Castro closed the casinos and threw out or imprisoned leading Mafia figures. Jack Ruby is known to have visited such individuals in Castro's prisons.

The Vice-President at that time, Richard Nixon, was put in charge of CIA efforts to overthrow Castro and install a government more favorable to

---

* In a deathbed confession Hunt told his son that the purpose of the Watergate break-in was to retrieve documents from a safe that linked Nixon to Operation 40 and the Kennedy assassination. Operation 40 was a CIA sponsored paramilitary operation to train Cuban exiles for the overthrow of Fidel Castro.

the U.S.. Nixon thus had direct contact with CIA operatives and developed a first hand familiarity with CIA personnel, methods, and ongoing operations.

Nixon lost the 1960 election to Kennedy and became a Wall Street lawyer. He resurfaced at a party thrown by Texas oil millionaire Clint Murchison in Dallas the night before the assassination. Also in attendance were J. Edgar Hoover and Lyndon Johnson.

Nixon was elected President a few years later in 1968, and re-elected in 1972. Nixon's Vice President, Spiro Agnew, resigned in disgrace in 1973 amid charges that he engaged in corrupt practices while Governor of Maryland. Nixon then appointed former Warren Commissioner Gerald Ford as his new Vice President. It was Ford who rewrote the final Warren Commission Report to reposition Kennedy's back wound up into his neck to facilitate Arlen Specter's magic bullet theory. A month after Nixon was forced to resign, Ford made the unusual move of pardoning Nixon for all crimes he may have committed while President.

Groden and Livingstone uncover other links between the Kennedy assassination, Nixon, and Watergate. Warren Commission Assistant Counsel David Belin was head of Lawyers for Nixon-Agnew. He was later appointed head of the Rockefeller Commission's investigation of intelligence activities, which examined the potential involvement of intelligence agencies in the murder of President Kennedy. No connection was found. Belin also conducted an investigation into allegations that E. Howard Hunt was involved in the President's assassination. No connection was found.

As the Watergate scandal started to unravel, Nixon's staff attempted to recruit J. Lee Rankin, General Counsel to the Warren Commission, as Special Prosecutor. Rankin also served as the Commission's liaison with the FBI and CIA. It was Rankin who cut off further debate on Arlen Specter's single bullet theory, later discredited as impossible. Nixon himself asked Arlen Specter to head his legal defense team, but was turned down.

It was Nixon's Attorney General, John Mitchell, who ordered the Justice Department to block release of the spectrographic analysis of the bullet and bullet fragments recovered from President Kennedy and Governor Connally after the assassination. The analysis would have determined if the bullet and all of the fragments had the same chemical composition, which would be required if Oswald was the lone sniper and the source of all of the bullets fired at the President. The analysis eventually disappeared from the

National Archives

Groden and Livingstone also detail numerous other Kennedy assassination items that have disappeared from the National Archives:

1. The President's brain, which had been deposited in the National Archives after the autopsy.

2. Color photographs of the President's chest taken at autopsy.

3. FBI laboratory technical records concerning spectrographic analysis of the ballistics evidence.

4. An FBI laboratory report concerning examination of the Presidential limousine.

5. A letter from Dallas Police Captain Will Fritz to the Warren Commission, dated June 9, 1964, concerning spent shells found at the Book Depository.

6. Warren Commission documentation for the "Records of the Dallas Police and County Sheriff's Office concerning arrests on November 22, 1963", and a photograph of suspect Jim Braden being arrested.

7. The official copy of the Dallas Police dictabelt recording of the shots fired at the President.

8. Tape recordings of Dallas Police Department radio broadcasts.

9. Two reports dealing with operational security at Oswald's transfer in the Dallas Police Headquarters.

10. A letter from the Commission to Dallas Police Lieutenant Jack Revill asking for records relating to Oswald and a pro-Castro demonstration.

11. The original statement of David Ferrie as transcribed in Commission Document 205.

12. A letter written by Warren Commission Assistant Counsel David Belin to Warren Commission General Counsel J. Lee Rankin on January 23, 1964, concerning the interrogation of Oswald by the Dallas Police Department.

13. A memorandum from Warren Commission Assistant Counsel Burt Griffin to J. Lee Rankin in August 1964 concerning unidentified fingerprints found on cartons at the Book Depository.

14. A 60 page memorandum from Warren Commission Assistant Counsel Joseph Ball and David Belin concerning the identity of the assassin.

15. A draft chapter for the Warren Commission Report submitted by Joseph Ball and David Belin in June 1964.

16. Two letters from Warren Commission Special Counsel Leon Jaworski to the Commission.

17. A letter from Warren Commissioner Gerald Ford on April 7, 1964 concerning expediting the FBI investigation.

High Treason also discusses the President's wounds as recorded at autopsy, and their divergence from the X-rays and pictures that were eventually produced by federal officials to support the idea that President Kennedy was hit by only two bullets fired from the sixth floor of the Texas School Book Depository, and that Oswald was the lone, unaided assassin. In fact, Groden and Livingstone demonstrate that the autopsy photographs and X-rays don't even agree with each other, with the photographs showing the President's face intact, and the X-rays showing the entire upper right front of his face blown off.

Groden and Livingstone ultimately conclude that Kennedy was killed in a carefully planned military style ambush set up by elements of the extreme right wing, the military-industrial complex, and the Mafia. They believe that the circle of conspirators was relatively small, but had the power of government and Mafia violence at their disposal. The conspirators were drawn to oppose Kennedy for his record on civil rights, his opposition to escalating the war in Vietnam, and his failure to seize Cuba from Castro. The destruction of evidence and the killing and intimidation of witnesses that followed the assassination were all designed to create a pattern of deliberate misinformation and confusion about what actually occurred on November 22, 1963.

CHAPTER 6

THEORIES OF THE ASSASSINATION

There is a multitude of theories about who killed President Kennedy and their motivation behind the assassination:

1. The Warren Commission: President Kennedy was shot by a lone deranged sniper named Lee Harvey Oswald. The President was struck by two bullets. Oswald shot the President to become famous, and acted alone. Oswald was then killed by Jack Ruby following a lapse in security at Dallas Police Headquarters. Ruby acted alone. Ruby had no substantial connection to organized crime. [1-3]

2. The House Select Committee on Assassinations: President Kennedy was probably killed as the result of a conspiracy that could have included members of anti-Castro groups and / or organized crime, acting as individuals. The President was struck by two bullets. Ruby had extensive connections to organized crime. [4]

3. The Mafia: The assassination of President Kennedy was a "Mob hit" carried out in its totality by elements of organized crime. The motivation was to put an end to prosecution by federal authorities and revenge for a perceived betrayal by the Kennedys, who attained the White House in 1960 with assistance from the Mafia. Organized crime stood to lose millions if their Havana gambling and prostitution operations remained shuttered by Fidel Castro. Mafia figures Jack Ruby, Carlos Marcello, and Santos Trafficante all exhibited advance knowledge that the President was going to be killed. Santos Trafficante in particular stated before the assassination that "Kennedy's not going to make the election. He's going to be

119

hit." [5] One variant of this theory includes the loss of illicit profits from heroin trafficking operations in Southeast Asia that would have occurred following a withdrawal from Vietnam. [6]

4. Big Oil and the Military Industrial Complex: President Kennedy was killed to preserve the economic interests of various groups who stood to lose millions of dollars with a continued Kennedy presidency. Big Oil would lose millions due to the loss of the federal oil depletion allowance, and the Military Industrial Complex was destined for major economic losses if Kennedy withdrew from involvement in Vietnam.

5. The Soviets: Lee Harvey Oswald was brainwashed by Soviet authorities during his stay in the Soviet Union. He returned home as a programmed "Manchurian Candidate" assassin to kill the President.

6. Fidel Castro and Cuba: Fidel Castro became aware of CIA-inspired plots to murder him, and sent assassins to the United States to kill the President.

7. The CIA: Disaffected elements within the CIA organized the assassination as revenge for Kennedy's refusal to provide military support for the failed Bay of Pigs invasion of Cuba, as well as Kennedy's dismissal of top CIA officials following the debacle. Kennedy was also planning a major reorganization of the agency to conform to its original charter as a foreign intelligence gathering operation.

8. Johnson and Hoover: The assassination was organized by Lyndon Johnson and J. Edgar Hoover to preserve and enhance their political power. Johnson viewed Kennedy as an obstacle to attaining the Presidency, and at the time of the assassination he appeared headed for a jail cell as the result of various scandals. J. Edgar Hoover was at the mandatory federal retirement age, and feared the loss of his job if Kennedy was reelected President in 1964. [7, 8]

These theories are not mutually exclusive. Many believe that the operational aspects of the assassination involved elements of both the CIA and organized crime, groups that were intertwined in their efforts to pry Cuba from the grip of Fidel Castro.

As shown in Chapters 1 - 3, however, dark forces within the federal government have quite openly conspired to alter the medical evidence to disguise the true nature of the President's wounds, namely that the President was struck by more than two bullets. As a result, the President's neck was not dissected at autopsy, based on a directive from a high ranking military official present at the autopsy. As a result, the President's brain was not properly sectioned, and in fact later disappeared. As a result, the autopsy team pretended that the President's back wound was in his neck. As a result, the Warren Commission concocted a bizarre single bullet scenario that could not possibly be true. As a result, phony pictures and X-rays appeared in the National Archives that did not in any way correspond to the written observations of the Parkland doctors, the Secret Service, the autopsy team, or the evidence published in the Warren Commission Report, all with nary a peep from government panel physicians or the press.

None of this could have been accomplished by the Mafia, the Soviet Union, Fidel Castro, Big Oil, or the Military Industrial Complex. It could only have been done by insiders within the federal government, leading to an inevitable conclusion:

> President Kennedy was assassinated as the result of a conspiracy that emanated, wholly or in part, from within the federal government of the United States. There is no other reason why employees of the federal government would attempt to cover up such a massive crime.

Any theory of the assassination that does not include the influence of the federal insiders who covered up this crime is destined to failure.

CHAPTER 7

THE THIRD IMPULSE: THE SHOT THAT KILLED THE PRESIDENT AND WOUNDED GOVERNOR CONNALLY

In any conspiracy an array of threats, real or implied, may be deployed to generate a desired outcome. These can include death threats, threats of physical harm to self and family, threats of property damage, threats to career, threats of financial ruin, and threats of malicious or false prosecution and possible jail time.

This is surely the case with the Kennedy assassination. Not only did many witnesses meet a violent end, there were numerous examples of how the FBI and Warren Commission used coercive tactics to shape witness testimony to arrive at the preordained conclusion that President Kennedy was hit by two bullets fired by a lone, unaided sniper.

In examining an event such as the Kennedy assassination the most trustworthy information often arrives at the beginning of the investigation, before the strategy and methods of intimidation can set in and alter the outcome. As a result, the best place to start is with the four wounds that were officially documented at Parkland Hospital and by the autopsy pathologists as of midnight, November 22, 1963:

1. A small, shallow entrance wound five inches down the back, just to the right of the spine and two inches deep; the bullet entered the back at an angle of approximately 45 to 60 degrees.

2. A small entrance wound at the base of the skull, just above the

occipital protuberance and an inch to the right of the midline.

3. A small wound at the front of the throat at the midline, just below the Adam's apple.

4. A large wound in the upper right quadrant of the head, extending across the top and back of the head.

These are the wounds that need to be explained by any scenario claiming a legitimate understanding of how the President was shot. The Warren Commission lacks credibility because it openly attempts to shoehorn these established facts into the predetermined conclusion that the President was struck by only two bullets. Any credible examination of the President's wounds must start without preconception as to how the wounds occurred and arrive at the most plausible explanation based on the observable facts.

As shown in Chapters 1 - 3, both of the President's entrance wounds have undergone a remarkable transformation from 1963 to 1979 in terms of their location and the scenarios used to explain them. By 1979 the federal government had produced the Report of the House Select Committee on Assassinations, in which it was claimed that all three autopsy pathologists were completely mistaken about the President having a wound at the base of his skull.

Instead the Committee asserted that a photograph in the National Archives shows a bullet wound at the top of the President's head, four inches higher than determined at autopsy, and that the back of the President's head was completely intact and undamaged, unlike the large gaping hole reported by the doctors at Parkland Hospital, Secret Service staff, the autopsy pathologists, and the Warren Commission. The Committee's report insinuated that the three autopsy pathologists, including a military wounds expert, were all completely fooled into thinking that there was a bullet hole at the base of the President's skull because of an extraneous piece of dried brain matter in his hair. It is of significance to note that the autopsy pathologists had access to developed X-rays of the President's skull at the time of the autopsy.

Author Harrison Livingstone has shown that the alleged entrance wound at the top of the President's head doesn't appear in other National Archives autopsy photographs showing the President's back, suggesting that it was added after the autopsy. [1]

In his testimony before the House Select Committee on Assassinations, Commander Humes made it clear that he observed and recorded an entrance wound at the base of the President's skull, and that this was the only entrance wound in the President's head. He went on to recount how he verified the location of the entrance wound by examining the President's skull from the inside after the brain had been removed. Figure 7-1 shows a laboratory specimen initialed by the autopsy pathologists at the location of the entrance wound just above the occipital protuberance of the skull.

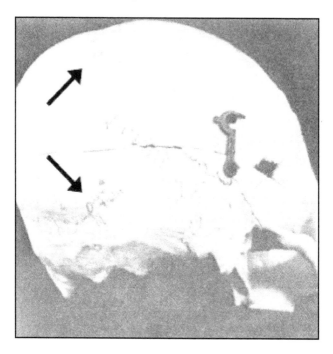

Figure 7-1. Laboratory skull initialed by the autopsy pathologists for the House Select Committee to document the location of the entrance wound at the base of the President's skull (lower arrow). The upper arrow shows the location of the same wound as specified by the Committee in 1979.

Figure 7-2 shows a reconstruction of the President's assassination performed by the FBI for the Warren Commission. The location of the President's entry wounds, including the shot to the base of the skull, are shown on the stand-in for the President.

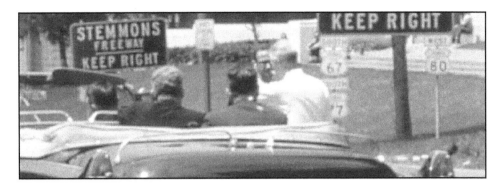

Figure 7-2. Reconstruction of the President's assassination performed by the FBI for the Warren Commission. The President's entry wounds are shown on the stand-in for the President, one at the base of his skull and the other five inches down his back.

From the outset it was well established that President Kennedy had been struck at the base of his skull. The November 24, 1963 edition of the New York Times carried an article by Dr. Howard A. Rusk entitled "The Kennedy Wound", and subtitled "Fatal Shot Struck Base of His Skull, Causing Immediate Unconsciousness". In the article Dr. Rusk states that "A high-velocity bullet that ripped through the base of the skull tore away the bone and brain tissue, striking the vital areas of the brain, the pons and medulla that control and regulate the vital functions of respiration and circulation." [2] *

Although it is clear that the autopsy pathologists determined that the President had an entrance wound at the base of his skull, their explanation of the resulting damage is transparently faulty.

The Warren Commission's published finding was that President Kennedy was killed by a shot fired from a height of six stories that entered the base of his skull and exploded out of the top of his head. The Commission produced a diagram showing the President leaning forward at such a steep angle that

---

* The brainstem is composed of three structures. These are, in ascending order from the spinal cord, the medulla oblongata, the pons, and the midbrain. The brainstem is also the origin of the reticular formation that controls the state of wakefulness throughout the brain. [3] Destruction of the brainstem would have resulted in instantaneous unconsciousness and death for the President.

he was facing the floor of his limousine (Figure 7-3A). The Zapruder film shows that this did not happen, and that the Warren Commission version cannot be true – the President was never leaning forward sufficiently for a shot entering the base of his skull to have exploded out of the top of his head (Figure 7-3B).

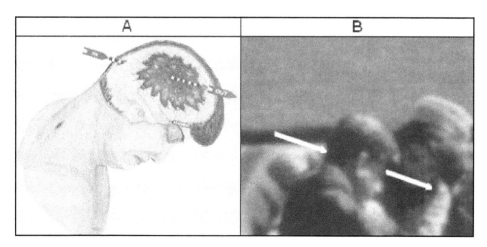

Figure 7-3. Warren Commission Exhibit 388 (A) showing the Commission's version of how a shot to the base of the President's skull exploded out of the top of his head, and (B) the President's actual position in Zapruder Frame 312, immediately before the "head shot" in Frame 313. Note that in the Commission's version the President was facing the limousine floor, when in fact he was almost upright. Zapruder Frame 312 shows that a bullet entering the base of the President's skull would have passed underneath the brain and exited at the level of the eyes.

Thus, to this day it remains unexplained what actually happened after the bullet struck the President at the base of his skull. If the Warren Commission's version is impossible, what actually occurred?

If one stands next to the sixth floor sniper's nest in Dallas and looks out of the window down at Elm Street (Figure 5-6), the solution to the riddle of the President's wounds becomes apparent. The sniper was six floors up and shooting down at the President. With the President sitting upright any shot striking the base of his skull and travelling in a straight line would exit the front of his neck (Figure 7-4).

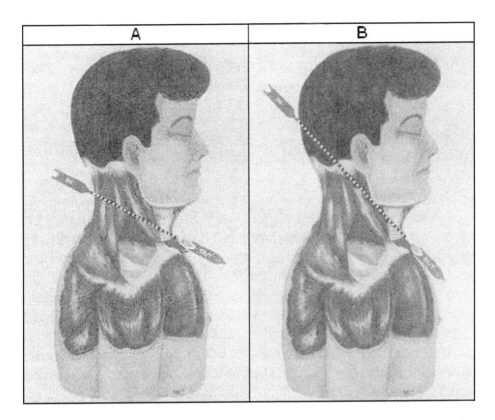

Figure 7-4. Redrawn versions of Warren Commission Exhibit 385 showing a bullet passing through the President at angles of 25 degrees (A) and 45 degrees (B). The angle shown at the left is the angle of declination* from the sixth floor sniper's nest - the point of entry is just below the wound shown in the FBI reconstruction depicted in Figure 7-2. The angle shown at the right is the same angle as the shot that entered the President's back - the point of entry is just above the entrance wound shown on the official autopsy face sheet (Figure 1-2).

---

* The term "angle of declination" refers to the rate of descent of the bullet, i.e. the distance that the bullet moves vertically relative to the distance that the bullet moves horizontally.

THE FIRST SHOT TO STRIKE THE PRESIDENT: THE MISFIRE

As murders go, the killing of President Kennedy is remarkably well documented. There is a frame by frame video account, a substantial photographic record, and acoustic data that pinpoint the exact spacing of the shots in time. When combined with the speed of the limousine, and knowledge of the exact point where the President's skull was shattered, the position of the President for each shot can be determined.

If one adopts the Warren Commission's view that shots were fired from the Texas School Book Depository, the shooter was six stories up, and shooting down at a substantial angle. Once the President's position on Elm Street is calculated for each shot, the exact angle of declination is known, and when combined with witness testimony and anatomic data yields a characteristic picture of how events unfolded.

At autopsy the pathologists found that a bullet had entered the President's back at an angle of 45 to 60 degrees, penetrating to a depth of approximately two inches. The autopsy pathologists thought that the bullet was subsequently dislodged as a result of efforts to resuscitate the President and was then recovered from a stretcher. This bullet eventually became Warren Commission Exhibit 399.

The steep angle at which the bullet entered indicates that it was one of the first shots fired at the President as he moved past the Dallas School Book Depository and down Elm Street. The Zapruder film shows the President waving to the crowd up to the point where his limousine starts to disappear behind a large traffic sign, and when he emerges from behind the sign he is clearly in serious distress. Both of his hands are tightly bunched in a fist and are beginning to rise (Figure 7-8).

Many believe that as the President emerges from behind the sign the upward movement of his fists indicates that he is voluntarily clutching at a wound in his throat. This is the case with Warren Commission supporters as well as conspiracy theorists.

Both the Warren Commission and House Select Committee claimed that a bullet entered the President's back and exited his throat. Conspiracy theorists generally believe that the anterior throat wound was an entrance wound created by a shot from the front. Both of these scenarios generally conclude that as the President emerges from behind the sign he is reacting to a wound in his throat, and that he is voluntarily attempting to move his hands up to that wound.

This, however, is a misconception. The visual record shows that the President was not voluntarily clutching at his throat, but rather reacting reflexly to the shot in his back. Figure 7-11 shows the position of the President's bunched hands in Zapruder Frame 236. It is clear that his hands continue to rise well above his throat until they are roughly in front of his forehead, still tightly bunched.

A number of physicians have identified this as the "Thornburn position", a reflex that occurs in cases of serious injury to the spine. [4-6]

There are two additional characteristics of the President's back wound that are unique: first, the bullet traveled a distance of only two inches after striking the President, hardly characteristic of military ordinance, and second, in most scenarios this bullet eventually came to be known as Warren Commission Exhibit (CE) 399.

The FBI matched CE 399 to the Mannlicher-Carcano rifle found on the sixth floor of the School Book Depository. A controversy then arose about the type of bullets used by the sixth floor sniper. In an Appendix entitled "Speculations and Rumors" the Warren Commission asserted:

Speculation. – Ammunition for the rifle found on the sixth floor of the Texas School Book Depository had not been manufactured since the end of World War II. The ammunition used by Oswald must, therefore, have been at least 20 years old, making it extremely unreliable.

Commission Finding. – The ammunition used in the rifle was American ammunition recently made by the Western Cartridge Company, which manufactures such ammunition currently. In tests with the same kind of ammunition, experts fired Oswald's Mannlicher-Carcano rifle more than 100 times without any misfires. [7]

Author Mark Lane, however, produced a letter dated July 14, 1965 from an Assistant Sales Service Manager at the Western Cartridge Division of Olin Mathieson Chemical Corporation, stating:

"Concerning your inquiry on the 6.5 millimeter Mannlicher-Carcano cartridge, this is not being produced commercially by our company at this time.

Any previous production on this cartridge was made against Government contracts which were completed back in 1944.

Therefore, any of this ammunition which is on the market today is Government surplus ammunition." [8]

This suggests that the ammunition used by the sixth floor sniper was old, unreliable and therefore prone to misfire. This would account for the weak penetration of the missile into President Kennedy's back.

The angle of declination from the sixth floor sniper's nest to the point on Elm Street where the President was first struck is approximately 25 degrees. The autopsy pathologists found, however, that the shot entered the President at an angle of 45 to 60 degrees. The difference could be attributed to the seating accommodations of the Presidential limousine. As shown in Figure 7-5, the back seat in which the President was riding had an expansive slope backwards, which would substantially increase the angle at which a shot fired from above and behind would enter the body. The President's seating arrangement could easily have added 20 degrees to the angle at which the bullet entered his back.

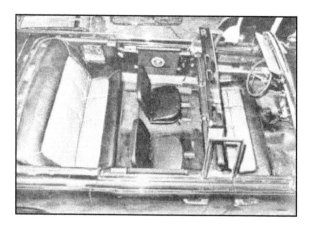

Figure 7-5. Warren Commission Exhibit 346: Interior of the Presidential limousine.

Consistent with the pathologists' statements at autopsy, one can therefore conclude that the first shot to strike the President was a shot from above and behind that lodged in his back, became dislodged during resuscitation efforts, and was subsequently discovered on a hospital stretcher. From there it eventually became CE 399.

THE SECOND SHOT TO STRIKE THE PRESIDENT: THE ASSASSIN'S SHOT

The President's autopsy found that the bullet that struck the President in the back entered at an angle of approximately 45 degrees. It was also determined that there was an entrance wound at the base of the President's skull, and an exit wound at the front of his throat, just below the Adam's apple. If a line is drawn at a 45 degree angle from the base of the skull, it will pass through the brainstem and exit the front of the throat, just below the Adam's apple (Figure 7-4B). A rifle shot following this path would have killed the President instantly.

A shot to the base of the skull is the shot that a professional assassin would use to eliminate a human target with certainty. A bullet entering the base of the skull and passing through the brainstem will kill instantly with one hundred percent efficiency.

Despite its obvious nature, this idea has not been given any consideration due largely to ideological factors: Warren Commission supporters believe that only two shots struck the President, and that the shot that struck the base of his skull exited the top of his head. Conspiracy theorists generally believe that the President's frontal throat wound was an entrance wound, indicative of a shot from the front.

While the idea that the President was hit by a shot that entered the base of his skull and exited his throat has received little public attention, it did make an appearance buried in the appendices of the Report of the House Select Committee on Assassinations.

The House Select Committee on Assassinations determined that two additional individuals had attended the autopsy, but were not on the list assembled by FBI agents Sibert and O'Neill: Samuel Bird, a lieutenant stationed at the ceremonial duties office at Fort Meyers, Virginia, and Richard Lipsey, a personal aide to General Wehle. The House Select Committee report contained the following:

"...staff interview with Richard A. Lipsey, Jan. 18, 1978, House Select Committee on Assassinations (JFK Document No. 014469), in which Lipsey stated that he recalled the doctors concluding that three missiles struck the President from behind. Lipsey said that one bullet entered the upper back of the President and did not exit; one entered in the rear of the head and exited the throat; and one entered and exited in the right, top portion of the head, causing a massive head wound.

The committee agreed that President Kennedy suffered a wound in the upper back, a wound in the rear of the head, a massive wound in the top, right side of the head, and a wound in the throat. Lipsey was wrong, however, in concluding that three shots struck the President and mistaken if he believed the pathologists reached such a conclusion. Only two shots struck the President: One entered the upper back and exited the throat. Another entered the rear of the head and exited the top, right side of the head, causing the massive defect.

Lipsey apparently formulated his conclusions based on observations and not on the conclusions of the doctors. In this regard, he believed the massive defect in the head represented an entrance and exit when it was only an exit. He also concluded that the entrance in the rear of the head corresponded to an exit in the neck. This conclusion could not have originated with the doctors, because during the autopsy they believed the neck defect only represented a tracheostomy incision. Lipsey did properly relate the preliminary conclusion of the doctors during the autopsy that the entrance wound in the upper back had no exit. The doctors later determined that this missile had exited through the throat. Thus, although Lipsey's recollection of the number of defects to the body and the corresponding locations are correct, his conclusions are wrong and are not supported by any other evidence." [9] *

The belief by conspiracy theorists that the President was hit in the throat by a shot from the front rests on two factors: first, the wound was small, and second, exit wounds are generally larger than entrance wounds, in some cases by a substantial margin.

The Parkland Hospital doctors initially estimated the size of the frontal throat wound to be about 5 millimeters, and stated that they thought the wound was an entrance wound. When the President arrived at the hospital he was bleeding profusely from a large head wound, and it appeared that he was about to die without rapid intervention. Little attention was paid to the throat wound and it was quickly obliterated by a required tracheotomy. It therefore received only the briefest of attention and examination.

During the subsequent investigation, the doctors revised the estimated size to 5 – 8 millimeters, and suggested that the wound could also have been an exit wound. Test results presented to the Warren Commission showed goatskin gunshot exit wounds that were only slightly larger than the corresponding entrance wounds. [10]

It is also evident that problems may arise when comparing an exit wound of the throat to an exit wound of the skull. When a supersonic bullet passes through a closed vessel such as the skull, it creates a large vacuum behind it as it rapidly displaces the material in its path. On exit this vacuum creates an explosive force outward.

The situation is not the same in the neck. When a bullet traverses the neck, much of its path is through unpressurized air, either in the esophagus or the trachea (windpipe). A bullet travelling from back to front near the midline would strike the inside wall of the trachea, in an open airway, just before exiting the neck. This would give the resulting frontal throat wound an appearance more like the inside edge of an entrance wound, than, for example, the large hole generated by the explosive outward force of an exit wound of the skull.

---

* This passage clearly illustrates the whitewash inclinations of the House Select Committee with regard to the medical evidence. Instead of giving Lipsey's scenario serious consideration, the Committee chose to unquestioningly stand behind the single bullet theory, which is contradicted by a mountain of evidence.

Another factor to be considered is that the tissue of the anterior surface of the throat possesses elastic properties that the skull does not. This elasticity will allow the surface to deform considerably, allow a bullet to pass, and then snap back into place. Moreover, a shot from the front using military grade ordinance would have resulted in substantially more damage to the President's neck than was evident. Except for the spinal column, the neck consists largely of soft tissue and the unpressurized airspace of the esophagus and trachea. If a frontal bullet missed the spinal column it surely would have exited, and if it had struck the spinal column, the President would have been effectively decapitated. Neither event occurred.

It is therefore reasonable to conclude that the Warren Commission's assertion that the President's frontal throat wound was an exit wound is entirely plausible.

Evidence that a shot entered the base of the President's skull and transected his brainstem can be found in the testimony of Dr. Humes before the forensic pathology panel of the House Select Committee. The forensic pathology panel discussed substantial damage to structures near the brainstem on the underside of the brain. Dr. Humes noted that "the midbrain was virtually torn from the pons" and that the damage was "partly caused by the bullet". [11]

At autopsy the brain must be severed from the spinal cord for the brain's removal from the skull, but another of the autopsy pathologists, Dr. Boswell, maintained that the President's brain was quite easily removed from the skull without recourse to surgery. [12] Boswell's remarks indicate that the brain did not have to be cut from the spinal cord, suggesting that the spinal cord was already severed as a result of the President's injuries.

The idea that a bullet hit the President at the base of his skull, obliterated his brainstem, and then exited his throat simply connects the dots established by the Warren Commission. According to the Commission the President had an entrance wound at the base of his skull and an exit wound at the front of his throat. A bullet shot from a height of six stories striking the President at the base of the skull would have exited his throat. If the same bullet continued in a straight line, it would have struck Governor Connally in the back below his armpit and likely would have caused all of his wounds (Figure 7-6).

This scenario is in fact identical to the Warren Commission's single bullet theory, less the Commission's imaginary entrance wound in the neck, less the Commission's imaginary change of direction, and less the Commission's ridiculous idea that such a bullet could remain unfragmented and in pristine condition while leaving behind numerous fragments in Governor Connally.

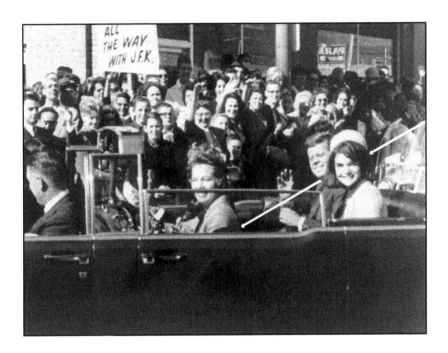

Figure 7-6. Photograph showing the relative vertical positioning of President Kennedy and the Connallys (at center). The Connallys were both seated on fold-up "jump seats" that were essentially bolted to the floor of the limousine (Figure 7-5), and were therefore about six inches lower than the Kennedys. A shot passing through the base of President Kennedy's skull at an angle of 29 degrees would have struck Governor Connally vertically at a level just below the armpit.

THE THIRD SHOT TO STRIKE THE PRESIDENT:
THE HEAD SHOT

Given the location and massive force that was applied by the third shot to strike the President, it appears that the injury could be described largely as a tangential wound, with no discernible entry or exit, extending from behind the right temple through the back of the head, with significant disruption evident throughout the top of the head (Figures 1-2 and 4-2A).

The salient question is whether the shot came from above and behind the President, as maintained by the Warren Commission and House Select Committee on Assassinations, or from the right front, in the area behind the fence overlooking the grassy knoll. The bulk of evidence favors a shot from the right front:

1. When the bullet struck the President, his head and torso were instantaneously rocketed back and to the left.

2. The doctors at Parkland Hospital, Secret Service staff, autopsy pathologists, and the Warren Commission found that the President had a large gaping hole in the back of his head, usually indicative of a shot from the front.

3. In testimony before the Warren Commission, Secret Service Agent Clint Hill stated that the right rear portion of the President's head was missing, and that "it was lying in the rear seat of the car". A shot from behind would have propelled the debris forward of the President's seat.

4. Debris from the President's wounds was deposited on the motorcycle officer to the left and in back of the President, leading him to dismount his motorcycle and run up the grassy knoll.

5. The Bolt, Beranek, and Newman acoustical analysis showed that a shot originated from a supersonic rifle to the right front of the President about the time he was hit.

6. There were numerous eyewitness and earwitness accounts of shots fired from the right front.

7. There was a strong odor of gunpowder around the grassy knoll; the sixth floor window of the Texas School Book Depository was

300 feet away.

8.   Many suspect that it was high ranking CIA employee E. Howard Hunt who was apprehended as one of the "Three Tramps" in the rail yard behind the grassy knoll. Hunt gave a deathbed confession to his participation in the assassination (Chapter 8). His apprehension behind the grassy knoll suggests the participation of elements of the CIA in engineering a strike on the President from that location.

One of the ultimate ironies of the assassination is that the head shot was completely unnecessary. The second shot to strike the President had already killed him. It inflicted an unsurvivable wound that rendered him unconscious instantaneously.

The head shot and the subsequent rapid backward thrust of the President's body have served historically as a stimulus for efforts to determine what really happened in Dealey Plaza on November 22, 1963.

Ironically, that shot was not necessary.

THE TIMING OF THE SHOTS

The summary acoustical data that Bolt, Beranek and Newman (BBN) used to draw their conclusions about the shots fired at President Kennedy are shown in Figure 7-7. [13]

The first column is time in seconds after the onset of the open motorcycle transmitter. The second column corresponds to the position of each microphone on Elm Street.

In refining their analysis for the impulse times at 137.70, 139.27, 145.15, and 145.61 seconds, BBN selected the data whose microphone position had the best match to the estimated position of the motorcycle at the time of the shooting.

However, BBN excluded the data for the third impulse at 140.32 seconds (shown by the arrow in Figure 7-7) solely because the timing of the shot was too close to the previous impulse at 139.27 seconds, and could not have been generated by the same sixth floor shooter in that brief interval. [14]

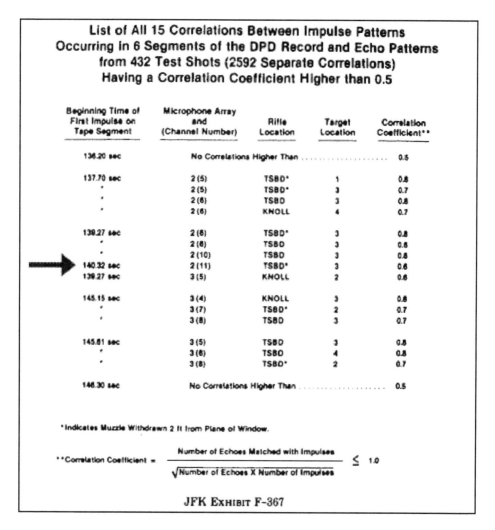

**List of All 15 Correlations Between Impulse Patterns
Occurring in 6 Segments of the DPD Record and Echo Patterns
from 432 Test Shots (2592 Separate Correlations)
Having a Correlation Coefficient Higher than 0.5**

Beginning Time of First Impulse on Tape Segment	Microphone Array and (Channel Number)	Rifle Location	Target Location	Correlation Coefficient**
136.20 sec	No Correlations Higher Than			0.5
137.70 sec	2 (5)	TSBD*	1	0.8
"	2 (5)	TSBD*	3	0.7
"	2 (6)	TSBD	3	0.8
"	2 (6)	KNOLL	4	0.7
139.27 sec	2 (6)	TSBD*	3	0.8
"	2 (6)	TSBD	3	0.6
"	2 (10)	TSBD	3	0.8
140.32 sec	2 (11)	TSBD*	3	0.6
139.27 sec	3 (5)	KNOLL	2	0.6
145.15 sec	3 (4)	KNOLL	3	0.8
"	3 (7)	TSBD*	2	0.7
"	3 (8)	TSBD	3	0.7
145.61 sec	3 (5)	TSBD	3	0.8
"	3 (6)	TSBD	4	0.8
"	3 (8)	TSBD*	2	0.7
146.30 sec	No Correlations Higher Than			0.5

*Indicates Muzzle Withdrawn 2 ft from Plane of Window.

$$**\text{Correlation Coefficient} = \frac{\text{Number of Echoes Matched with Impulses}}{\sqrt{\text{Number of Echoes X Number of Impulses}}} \leq 1.0$$

JFK Exhibit F-367

Figure 7-7. House Select Committee on Assassinations JFK Exhibit F-367 showing the summary data from Bolt, Beranek and Newman for the shots fired in Dealey Plaza.

The exclusion of the third impulse assumes that there was not another shooter situated in the vicinity of the sniper's nest on the sixth floor of the Dallas School Book Depository. This is certainly not a valid assumption - there could easily have been more than one shooter firing at the President from that area. As it turns out, the third impulse is the key to understanding what actually occurred on November 22, 1963.

The BBN analysis concluded that the impulse at 145.15 came from the grassy knoll. If the assumption is made that this corresponds to the "head shot" in Zapruder Frame 313, the corresponding Zapruder frames can be calculated.

Using the impulse at 137.70 seconds as the first shot at time zero, and a Zapruder frame rate of 18.3 frames / second, this yields:

Impulse #1: Time = 0.00 seconds, Zapruder Frame = 177

Impulse #2: Time = 1.57 seconds, Zapruder Frame = 205

Impulse #3: Time = 2.62 seconds, Zapruder Frame = 225

Impulse #4: Time = 7.45 seconds, Zapruder Frame = 313

Impulse #5: Time = 7.91 seconds, Zapruder Frame = 321

The BBN data were further refined by Professors Weiss and Aschkenasy to correct an error in tape recorder speed and variability in the speed of Zapruder's movie camera, yielding the more familiar values of 0.00, 1.66, 7.49, and 8.31 seconds for impulses 1, 2, 4, and 5. It should be noted that the BBN values in Figure 7-7 are the impulses as recorded directly into an open police microphone in Dealey Plaza, whereas the Weiss and Aschkenasy values are the estimated trigger pull times. A memorandum from Chief Counsel Blakey explaining this procedure is contained in Appendix B.

If the third impulse at 140.32 seconds in Figure 7-7 is interpolated into the Weiss and Aschkenasy sequence, the result is 0.00, 1.66, 2.70, 7.49, and 8.31 seconds. If the shot from the grassy knoll is used to anchor the data to Zapruder Frame 313, the corresponding Zapruder Frames are 176, 206, 225, 313, and 328.

In either sequence (original Dallas Police Department tape or the Weiss and Aschkenasy sequence), the Zapruder frame is the same for the third impulse (225), although it is necessary to add two additional Zapruder frames to the Weiss and Aschkenasy interpolation to account for the time it would take for a bullet to travel from the weapon to the target. This yields a target strike in Zapruder Frame 227.

The Dallas Police determined that during the shooting a spectator named James Tague was standing near the underpass at the far end of Elm Street and was wounded by a bullet ricochet off the curb close to the underpass. Any complete accounting of the shots fired at the President must include the wounding of Tague.

Although the Warren Commission was noncommittal as to which shot missed the President and hit Tague, most Warren Commission supporters believe that it was the first shot fired. While this may be convenient, it seems improbable. The President was less than 50 yards down Elm Street when the first shot was fired, so a miss at that point would have been by more than 100 yards. A more likely scenario is that Tague was hit toward the end of the sequence, when the Presidential limousine was further down Elm Street and at a flatter angle relative to the Texas School Book Depository.

There is little doubt that the first impulse at Zapruder Frame 177 corresponds to a shot that missed the President entirely. Most analyses indicate that the sixth floor sniper would have been shooting through a tree blocking his view.

The House Select Committee noted the presence of a girl running on the grass parallel to the motorcade. She suddenly stops running at about Zapruder Frame 186, then turns to look at the back of the motorcade. The Committee took this to be evidence of a possible shot being fired just before she stops running. [15]

Through Zapruder Frame 193 the President is waving to the crowd, but by Frame 198, just before a large traffic sign obscures the President, there is a noticeable change in posture and he has stopped waving. Many of the frames in this region evidence substantial blur, and it is not possible to get a clear look at the President's facial expression. While a change in the President's posture is evident, he does not appear to have been slammed forward. It is possible that he is reacting to the sound of the first shot.

By Zapruder Frame 206 the President has almost disappeared behind the sign, with just his head showing. The House Select Committee found that by Zapruder Frame 207 the President was reacting to a "severe external stimulus". [16] *

Governor Connally appears first as the limousine emerges from behind the traffic sign. Zapruder Frame 223 shows that he is his facing Zapruder's camera off to his right, and he appears to be sitting turned to the right with his right shoulder resting squarely on the back of his seat. President Kennedy emerges in Zapruder Frame 225, his fists clenched tight, starting

---

* Zapruder Frames 208 – 212 are unavailable for study because they are missing, allegedly due to a problem processing the film.

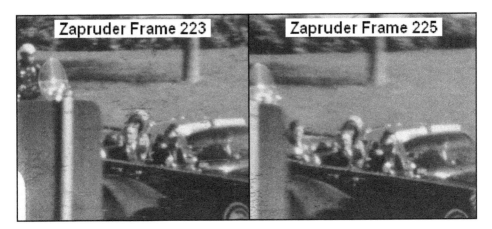

Figure 7-8. Zapruder Frames 223 and 225 showing Governor Connally and President Kennedy as they emerge from behind a large traffic sign. Note that the President's hands are already clenched tightly in a fist and rising from the spinal reflex induced by the shot in his back.

to rise upward (Figure 7-8).

Figure 7-9 shows President Kennedy and Governor Connally being slammed forward simultaneously in Zapruder Frame 227. A bullet has struck President Kennedy at the base of his skull, transected his brainstem, and exited from the front of his neck. The President is now dead. The bullet continues in a straight line to strike Governor Connally in the back, exiting his chest, and striking him in the wrist. The bullet disintegrates, leaving numerous fragments in Governor Connally, as well as two large fragments on the limousine floor.

The President continues to tightly clench his fists from the reflex induced by the bullet in his back (Figure 7-11). His fists continue to rise for about a second, reaching their zenith at Zapruder Frame 247. At this point the President's arms slowly begin to relax, and he slumps forward, dead, held up only by his back brace.

Three seconds later the upper right quadrant of the President's skull is removed by a shot from behind the grassy knoll, instantaneously rocketing the President back and to the left. The shot is unnecessary. The President is already dead.

The final shot misses the President, ricochets off the curb, and strikes spectator James Tague. The open police microphone records the last two shots as being less than a half second apart, and many in Dealey Plaza,

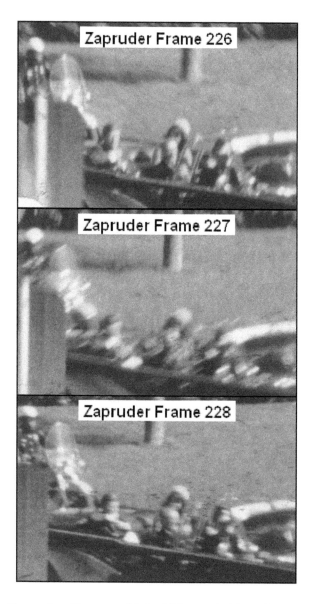

Figure 7-9. Zapruder Frames 226, 227, and 228 showing the frames before, during, and after President Kennedy and Governor Connally are both slammed forward simultaneously in Frame 227. Note the position of Governor Connally's head relative to Jacqueline Kennedy's head in Frames 226 – 228.

particularly those closer to the Dallas School Book Depository, will hear them merged as a single shot.

A summary of these events is shown in Figure 7-10.

Impulse Number	Trigger Pull Time	Zapruder Frame	EVENT
1	0.00	176	Missed shot.
2	1.66	206	Shot from above and behind hits the President 5 inches down his back and just to the right of his spine, corresponding to the location of the bullet holes in his shirt and suit jacket.
3	2.70	225	Shot from above and behind hits the President at the base of his skull and exits the front of his throat, killing him instantly; the shot continues in a straight line to strike Governor Connally.
4	7.49	313	Shot from the right front tangentially strikes the right side of the President's head and removes the upper right quadrant of his skull and underlying brain mass.
5	8.31	328	Missed shot, ricochet hits James Tague.

Figure 7-10. Account of the President's wounds assembled by interpolating the third impulse of the BBN data (Figure 7-7) into the "trigger pull time" analysis of Professors Weiss and Aschkenasy (Note: the Zapruder frames listed in Column 3 correspond to the trigger pull times in Column 2; the frame showing the actual bullet strike is typically 1–3 frames later, depending on the distance from the weapon to the target).*

---

* Shot #3 occurs only 1.04 seconds after Shot #2, eliminating the possibility that they were both fired from the same bolt action rifle. According to the BBN analysis, the shot came from the vicinity of the sixth floor sniper's nest, indicating that it came from above and behind the President

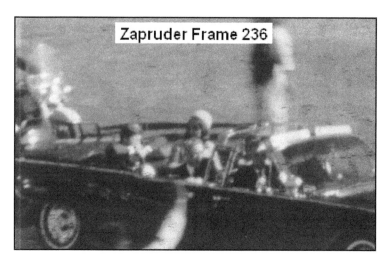

Figure 7-11. Governor Connally is shown grimacing in Zapruder Frame 236. Note that the President's hands are still tightly bunched in a fist and rising well above his throat, indicating that his movements were the result of an involuntary reflex from the shot to his back, and not a voluntary clutching at his throat.

WHERE DID THE FATAL SHOT COME FROM?

The Bolt, Beranek, and Newman analysis shown in Figure 7-7 indicates that the third impulse on the Dallas Police tape had the acoustic properties of a shot coming from the Texas School Book Depository. The previous impulse, however, occurs only 1.04 seconds before this shot, too close in time to have been generated by the same bolt action rifle. If the second impulse corresponds to the shot in the President's back, the third could not have come from the same bolt action Mannlicher-Carcano rifle that was eventually tied to Oswald and CE 399.

 There would have had to have been another shooter in the Texas School Book Depository.

Figures 7-12 and 7-13 show Dallas Police and FBI affidavits sworn by eyewitness Arnold Rowland, who states that he saw a man with a rifle standing behind the westernmost sixth floor window of the Texas School Book Depository. He assumed the man was in the Secret Service.

VOLUNTARY STATEMENT. Not Under Arrest. Form No. 88

SHERIFF'S DEPARTMENT
COUNTY OF DALLAS, TEXAS

Before me, the undersigned authority, on this the 22nd day of November A. D. 19 63

personally appeared Arnold Louis Rowland, Address 3026 Remmerly St., Dallas, Texas

[illegible] POB: Corpus Christi, Texas

Age ______, Phone No. FE 7 1251

Deposes and says:-

I am a student at Adamson High School in Dallas, Texas. I am employed on weekends at the Pizza Inn located on West Davis Avenue in Dallas. At approximately 12:10PM today, my wife Barbara and I arrived in downtown Dallas and took position to see the President's motorcade. We took position at the west entrance of the Sheriff's Office on Houston Street. We stood there for a time talking about various things and were talking about the security measures that were being made for the president's visit in view of the recent trouble when Mr. Adalai Stevenson had been a recent visitor to Dallas. It must have been 5 or 10 minutes later when we were just looking at the surrounding buildings when I looked up at the Texas Book Depository building and noticed that the second floor from the top had two adjoining windows which were wide open, and upon looking I saw what I thought was a man standing back about 15 feet from the windows and was holding in his arms what appeared to be a hi powered rifle because it looked as though it had a scope on it. He appeared to be holding this at a parade rest sort of position. I mentioned this to my wife and merely made the remark that it must be the secret service man. This man appeared to be a white man and appeared to have a light colored shirt on, open at the neck. He appeared to be of slender build and appeared to have dark hair. In about 15 minutes President Kennedy passed the ~~spxxx~~ spot where we were standing and the motorcade had just turned west on Elm heading down the hill when I heard a noise which I thought to be a back fire. In fact some of the people around laughed and then in about 8 seconds I heard another report and in about 3 seconds a third report. My wife, who had ahold, of my hand, started running and dragging me across the street and I never did look up again at this window.

This statement is true and correct to the best of my knowledge and belief.

Arnold L. Rowland

Subscribed and sworn to before me on this the 22nd day of November A. D. 19 63

Rosemary Allen

Notary Public, Dallas County, Texas

Commission Exhibit No. 357

55

Figure 7-12. Warren Commission Exhibit 357, a Dallas Police Affidavit by eyewitness Arnold Rowland.

"Dallas, Texas
November 24, 1963

"I, Arnold Louis Rowland, make the following statement of my own free will to James W. Swinford and Paul E. Wulff, who have identified themselves as Special Agents of the Federal Bureau of Investigation.

"I am 18 years of age, live at 3026 Hammerly, and am employed at Pizza Inn, 2841, West Davis, Dallas, Texas.

"My wife Barbara and I arrived at a point on Houston Street in Dallas between Main and Elm Streets at about 12:10 p.m., November 22, 1963, for the purpose of observing President Kennedy in the motorcade. The exact position where we were located was on the sidewalk on the west side of the Dallas County Courthouse just under the office of Sheriff Decker and a few feet to the south of the elevator shaft which comes out of the sidewalk.

"Between 12:10 p.m. and 12:15 p.m. , I looked toward the Texas School Book Depository which faces the South and is located on the corner of Elm and Houston. I observed the two rectangular windows at the extreme west end of the Texas School Book Depository on the next to the top floor were open. I saw what I believed to be a man standing about 12 to 15 feet back from the window on the right. He appeared to be slender in proportion to his height, was wearing a white or light colored shirt, either collarless or open at the neck. He appeared to have dark hair. He also appeared to holding a rifle with scope attached, in a ready position or in military terminology, port arms. I saw him only momentarily and he seemed to disappear in the shadows of the room.

/ at the time
"I gave this no further consideration as I believed he was probably a Secret Service man. I also called this to the attention of my wife, but she did not see the man.

"About 15 or 20 minutes later the President came by, but I did not see him get shot, nor did I see any shots fired. I did hear three shots. By about 1:45 p.m. I had advised an officer of what I had seen and I was taken to the Office of Sheriff Decker.

DL 89-43

"I would not be able to identify the person I saw due to the distance involved.

"I have read this 3-page statement which contains to my knowledge the correct truth.

"/s/ ARNOLD L. ROWLAND
11-24-63

"WITNESSES:

"/s/PAUL E. WULFF
"Special Agent, FBI, Dallas, Texas
"/s/JAMES W. SWINFORD,
"Special Agent, FBI, Dallas, Texas"

Figure 7-13. Warren Commission Exhibit 358, an FBI Affidavit by eyewitness Arnold Rowland.

146

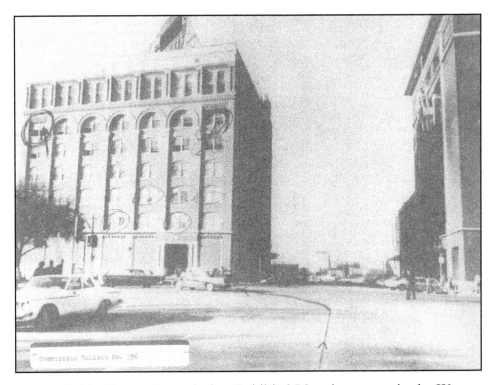

Figure 7-14. Warren Commission Exhibit 356 as it appears in the Warren Commission Report. The exhibit shows the Texas School Book Depository with both Oswald's alleged location and the westernmost sixth floor window at the left heavily circled. The sixth floor window at the left is where eyewitness Arnold Rowland saw a man standing with a rifle just before the assassination.

The window at which Rowland observed a man with a rifle was on the same floor as Oswald's alleged sniper's nest, but at the opposite end of the building. Figure 7-14 shows Warren Commission Exhibit 356, a photograph of the Texas School Book Depository with both the easternmost and westernmost sixth floor windows circled. The window at the upper left is where Rowland observed a man with a rifle. It is located roughly sixty feet closer to the President and therefore a shooter at that location would have been firing at a steeper angle than from the sniper's nest at the right. At Zapruder Frame 227 a shooter standing at that location would have been firing at the President at a 29 degree angle of declination. Figure 7-15 shows the path of a bullet striking the President at an angle of 29 degrees.

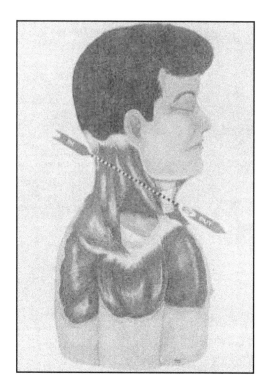

Figure 7-15. Redrawn version of Warren Commission Exhibit 385 showing a bullet passing through the President at 29 degrees, the unadjusted angle of declination from the westernmost sixth floor window of the Texas School Book Depository at Zapruder Frame 227. The point of entry is the same as that shown in the FBI reconstruction depicted in Figure 7-2. The point of exit is at the level of the Adam's apple.*

---

* There is no transcript or recording of Oswald's interrogation at Dallas Police Headquarters, but the Warren Commission Report contains an account by FBI Special Agents James Hosty and James Booxhout concerning Oswald's interrogation by Dallas Police Captain Will Fritz of the homicide bureau. Fritz asked Oswald if he ever owned a rifle. Oswald denied ever owning a rifle, but stated that he had observed Texas School Book Depository supervisor Roy Truly displaying a rifle in his office two days before the assassination. While Oswald's response could be considered self-serving, it does suggest the possibility that there was already a second rifle in the building at the time of the assassination. [17]

The President's autopsy noted that the wound at the base of the skull was just above the occipital protuberance and an inch to the right of the midline. The geometry of a shot from the westernmost window of the sixth floor of the Texas School Book Depository is consistent with entry an inch to the right of the midline and exit at the midline of the throat.

QUESTIONS WERE ASKED ABOUT THE HOUSE SELECT COMMITTEE VERSION

Questions have been raised about the acoustical data used by the House Select Committee. One of these concerns crosstalk on the original Dallas Police recording system, which was probably inevitable given the type of recording technology used in 1963.

Another concerns the type of statistical analysis used by Weiss and Aschkenasy to determine with 95% certainty that the shot at 7.49 seconds emanated from the grassy knoll.

Given the unique characteristics of the data, namely digitized acoustical echo profiles, questions about the statistical analysis and related conclusions are clearly legitimate because such specialty data require custom designed statistics that extend beyond those validated and used for general scientific experimentation. Statistical questions, however, do not negate the fact that the shots were spaced too closely together to have been fired by a single shooter using a bolt action rifle.

More recently a claim has been made that the shots on the Dallas Police tape are just random noise, or the sounds of a motorcycle, and that "the HSCA's analysis mistook individual features of unrelated sounds generated by vibrating, resonant objects for gunfire impulses." [18] Such an assertion shows a lack of understanding concerning the parameters being measured. The analyses by Bolt, Beranek, and Newman, and Professors Weiss and Aschkenasy, measured the return times for echoes off of the numerous large reflective surfaces in Dealey Plaza, which are unique for every combination of shooter position and microphone position. This generates a unique acoustical "fingerprint" for each combination (Figure 7-16). The idea that the Dallas Police recording consists of random sounds "generated by vibrating, resonant objects" that coincidentally match the echo profiles of shots in Dealey Plaza is beyond reasonable consideration.

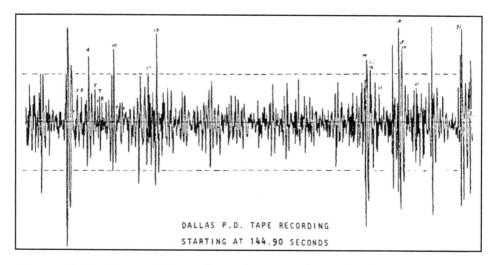

Figure 7-16. House Select Committee on Assassinations JFK Exhibit F-667, an oscillograph of the Dallas Police tape enumerating the spikes that correspond to echoes reflected off of large surfaces in Dealey Plaza. The timing of the spikes correlate to those observed for test shots fired in Dealey Plaza. The entire trace is 0.4 seconds in length.

Only four shots are necessary to fulfill the ballistics scenario described in this chapter – three shots striking the President and one shot striking James Tague – but use of the Dallas Police tape mandates that all five shots be taken into account, meaning inclusion of a fifth shot that missed completely.

The House Select Committee on Assassinations addressed this problem by simply removing one of the shots as a matter of convenience, but their justification for doing so – that the shot was too close in time to its predecessor – does not stand up to scientific or forensic scrutiny.

There are a number of factors that complicate analysis of how witnesses heard the shots in Dealey Plaza: i) the booming echo chamber environment of the plaza, with numerous large surfaces reflecting and refracting sound waves, ii) the constant backfiring of police motorcycles in the motorcade, iii) the pronounced investigative bias towards three shots, and iv) the three different physical locations of the shooters.

All of these factors complicate and confuse the perception and recall of shots arriving in rapid sequence without prior warning, particularly amidst the cacophony of police motorcycle backfires.

The evidence reveals that at the open police microphone the first three shots occurred within a span of 2.62 seconds, followed by a lull of 4.83 seconds, followed by the final two shots within 0.46 seconds of each other. The final two shots were less than a half second apart, and to the unpracticed, uneducated ear this would typically be heard as a single, merged shot, reducing the perceived total to four.

The backfiring of police motorcycles in the Presidential motorcade was a common occurrence in Dallas, and indeed many witnesses mistook the initial start of the shooting for police motorcycle backfires (see, for example, Figure 7-12). It was only after a period of time had elapsed that they realized that something more sinister was occurring. There was a continuous backfiring of police motorcycles throughout the motorcade, and in fact technical analysis of the police tape determined that the five shots were immediately preceded by an impulse that appears to have been a motorcycle backfire. [19] *

For fifty years the official and mainstream media account has been that three shots were heard in Dealey Plaza – three cartridges in the sniper's nest meant three shots at the President. The majority of witnesses in Dealey Plaza were documented by the FBI and the Warren Commission as having stated that they heard three shots.

Fourteen, however, said that they heard four or more shots. [21] Their testimony also shows how investigators used coercive tactics to shape witness testimony to conform to the three cartridges - three bullets - three shots narrative.

President Kennedy's Appointments Secretary Kenneth O'Donnell once confided to House Speaker Tip O'Neill that he had been pressured by the FBI to alter his testimony concerning the shots. O'Donnell said that "I told the FBI what I had heard, but they said it couldn't have happened that way and that I must have been imagining things. So I testified the way they wanted me to. I just didn't want to stir up any more pain and trouble for the family." [22]

In testimony before the Warren Commission witness Robert Edwards clearly felt pressured to say there were three shots, although he had heard four:

---

*A Bell Laboratories analysis of a radio station tape of the assassination found a short duration spike, followed by three longer duration sounds, and then another two longer duration sounds. [20]

Mr. Belin: How many shots did you hear, if you remember?

Mr. Edwards: Well, I heard one more then than was fired, I believe.

Mr. Belin: You mean you said on the affidavit you heard four shots?

Mr. Edwards: I still right now don't know how many was fired. If I said four, then I thought I heard four.

Mr. Belin: If you said four, you mean the affidavit – maybe we'd better introduce it into the record as Edward's Deposition Exhibit A...[23]

The House Select Committee uncovered an internal FBI report documenting the FBI's investigative bias during interviews with witnesses immediately after the assassination:

"According to that report (an FBI reinterview of Jean Hill [24] concerning her initial FBI interview on November 23, 1963 [25]), Mrs. Hill said that men who were either FBI or Secret Service agents were present later that afternoon when she was being questioned in the sheriff's office. Mrs. Hill related that one of the men referred to a bullet hitting the ground near her feet; she told him she did not recall such an incident. When she told the men that she had heard four to six shots, one of them said: 'There were three shots, three bullets, that's enough for now'." [26]

Hill was standing on Elm street with her friend Mary Moorman* at the point where Kennedy was hit. She told Warren Commission Assistant Counsel Arlen Specter exactly what she heard on November 22, 1963:

Mr. Specter: How many shots were there altogether?

Mrs. Hill: I have always said that there were some four to six shots. There were three shots – one right after the other, and a distinct

---

* Moorman took a famous Polaroid photo of the assassination.

pause, or just a moment's pause, and then I heard more.

Mr. Specter: How long a time elapsed from the first to the third of what you described as the first three shots?

Mrs. Hill: They were rapidly – they were rather rapidly fired. [27]

Several years later Hill related to author Jim Marrs how Specter had threatened her to try to get her to change her account of the number of shots. Specter told her that "we can make you look as crazy as Marguerite Oswald and everybody knows how crazy she is. We could have you put in a mental institution if you don't cooperate with us." [28]

Both Governor Connally and his wife Nellie thought that three bullets struck the occupants of the limousine. Three bullets striking the limousine, plus the wounding of James Tague, equals a minimum of four shots.* In testimony before the Warren Commission Governor Connally stated that "the thought immediately passed through my mind that there were either two or three people involved or more in this or someone was shooting with an automatic rifle." [30]

Mrs. Connally offered compelling Warren Commission testimony to support the idea that her husband was hit after President Kennedy was struck in the back. Mrs. Connally observed President Kennedy being hit first, causing his bunched fists to rise up toward his face. A short time afterward her husband was hit:

Mrs. Connally: In fact the receptions had been so good every place that I had showed much restraint by not mentioning something about it before.

I could resist no longer. When we got past this area I did turn to the President and said, "Mr. President, you can't say Dallas doesn't love you."

---

* William Sullivan, Hoover's third in command at the FBI, maintained that the President was hit by two shots and that Governor Connally was hit by a third shot.[29] This was also the FBI's finding in its initial report to the Warren Commission.

Then I don't know how soon, it seems to me it was very soon, that I heard a noise, and not being an expert rifleman, I was not aware that it was a rifle. It was just a frightening noise, and it came from the right.

I turned over my right shoulder and looked back, and saw the President as he had both hands at his neck.

Mr. Specter: And you are indicating with your own hands, two hands crossing over gripping your own neck?

Mrs. Connally: Yes; and it seemed to me there was – he made no utterance, no cry. I saw no blood, no anything. It was just sort of nothing, the expression on his face, and he just sort of slumped down.

Then very soon there was the second shot that hit John. As the first shot was hit, and I turned to look at the same time, I recall John saying, "Oh, no, no, no." Then there was a second shot, and it hit John, and as he recoiled to the right, just crumpled like a wounded animal to the right, he said, "My God, they are going to kill us all." [31]

CHAPTER 8

E. HOWARD HUNT, FRANK STURGIS, AND MARITA LORENZ

Everette Howard Hunt graduated from Brown University in 1940 and entered the United States Naval Academy in February 1941. During World War II he worked as an intelligence officer in China. He joined the CIA in 1949, shortly after its creation. He became CIA station chief in Mexico in 1950, and by 1960 he was directly involved in plots to overthrow Fidel Castro. Hunt resigned from the CIA in 1970, and in 1971 he joined the Nixon White House. He rose to fame as the mastermind of the bungled Watergate break-in, and served 33 months in prison. Nixon was recorded on his infamous tapes as stating, "This fellow Hunt, he knows too damned much." [1]

Hunt's son, St. John Hunt, used to look at pictures of the "Three Tramps", only to see his father's face staring back at him (Figure 5-7). He knew with certainty that his famed CIA spy father was in Dealey Plaza at the time of the President's assassination and was apprehended immediately afterward in the train yard behind the grassy knoll. [2]

On his deathbed E. Howard Hunt gave a written confession to St. John Hunt:

"E. Howard scribbled the initials 'LBJ,' standing for Kennedy's ambitious vice president, Lyndon Johnson. Under 'LBJ,' connected by a line, he wrote the name Cord Meyer. Meyer was a CIA agent whose wife had an affair with JFK; later she was murdered, a case

155

that's never been solved.* Next his father connected to Meyer's name the name Bill Harvey, another CIA agent;** also connected to Meyer's name was the name David Morales, yet another CIA man and a well-known, particularly vicious black-ops specialist.*** And then his father connected to Morales' name, with a line, the framed words 'French Gunman Grassy Knoll'." [3] ****

A few days later St. John Hunt received additional pages from his father: Cord Meyer had discussed the plot with David Atlee Phillips, who recruited Bill Harvey and Antonio Veciana. He also met with Oswald during his trip to Mexico City. Veciana met with Frank Sturgis and David Morales, and the plan was to kill JFK in Miami. LBJ changed the plan to Dallas. [9]

A more recent rendition of E. Howard Hunt's confession appeared on former Minnesota Governor Jesse Ventura's *Conspiracy Theory* television show. St. John Hunt reiterated that the assassination was supposed to have taken place in Miami, but was changed to Dallas. The elder Hunt said that the code name for the assassination was "The Big Event", and that it involved Operation 40, David Morales, and Frank Sturgis. He described himself as being a "bench warmer" for the plot, and that Lyndon Johnson

---

* Mary Pinchot Meyer's affair with JFK and her subsequent murder are recounted in the book *Mary's Mosaic* by Peter Janney

** Bill Harvey had been head of a CIA assassination unit codenamed ZR/RIFLE, before being removed in October 1962. He preferred to use Corsican killers instead of Sicilians because they were less traceable to the Mafia. [4] CIA counter-intelligence chief James Angleton served as the primary conduit to J. Edgar Hoover for Harvey's activities; Angleton had "enormously influential contacts" with Hoover. [5]

*** Morales died just days before he was scheduled to testify before the House Select Committee on Assassinations.

**** Many conspiracy theorists believe that the "French Gunman" was Michel Mertz (aka Jean Souetre), a well-known assassin for the French Connection heroin syndicate. CIA documentation declassified in 1995 identifies Mertz / Souetre as having been in Dallas on November 22, 1963, and expelled from the U.S. two days later. Others believe the "French Gunman" to be Corsican Mafia assassin Lucien Sarti. Sarti also figures prominently in various scenarios involving three Corsicans shooting at the President. [6-8]

[handwritten annotations: "True" next to first footnote; "True" next to second footnote; "False" next to third footnote]

[handwritten note at bottom: "2 gunmen @ Egyptian Restaurant (Campisi) (F)"]

"had an almost maniacal urge to become President. He regarded JFK as an obstacle to achieving that." [10]

Frank Sturgis, named by E. Howard Hunt as one of his assassination co-conspirators, achieved fame as a burglar who was apprehended at Watergate. Years earlier he had been recruited to assist Fidel Castro in his takeover of Cuba at a time when Castro was not viewed as an adversary of the United States. After Castro's rise to power, Sturgis was installed in 1959 as Cuba's "Superintendent of Games of Chance". Eventually Castro closed the casinos and arrested several key Mafia figures, including Jack Ruby's close friend, Lewis McWillie, who ran the Tropicana Casino. [11]

Sturgis was known to be associated with the Mafia, particularly the Santos Trafficante crime syndicate in Florida, and with Mafia plots to kill Castro, as well as CIA sponsored anti-Castro training camps in the southern U.S.. [12] near New Orleans

One of these plots is detailed in the pages of the House Select Committee on Assassinations report describing an October 18, 1960 FBI memo concerning Mafia boss Sam Giancana:

"During a recent conversation with several friends, Giancana stated that Fidel Castro was to be done away with shortly, said it would occur in November. Moreover, Giancana said he had already met with the would-be assassin on three occasions, the last meeting taking place on a boat docked at the Fontainbleu Hotel, Miami Beach. Giancana stated everything had been perfected for killing Castro and that the assassin had arranged with a girl, not further described, to drop a 'pill' in some drink or food of Castro." [13]

The girl mentioned in the FBI memo was German born Marita Lorenz, who had become Castro's mistress. In Cuba she was also an associate of Frank Sturgis (whom she knew at the time as Frank Fiorini). She later became involved with Sturgis in anti-Castro operations in the U.S., working at an Operation 40 training camp in the Florida Everglades. In early 1961 she met an individual at the camp who was introduced to her as Lee Harvey Oswald, who she came to know as "Ozzie".

In testimony before the House Select Committee Lorenz described a meeting at anti-Castro leader Orlando Bosch's house in which a trip to Dallas was announced, and maps of Dallas were produced and studied.

She thought that the purpose of the trip was to burglarize an armory to seize weapons for the anti-Castro effort. Lorenz testified that on November 16, 1963 she and Operation 40 figures Jerry Patrick Hemming, Pedro Diaz Lanz, Frank Sturgis, Orlando Bosch, "Ozzie" Oswald, and Guillermo and Ignacio Novo traveled in a two-car caravan to Dallas and stayed at a motel. The trip to Dallas lasted approximately two days, and included a substantial arsenal of weapons. She stated that at the motel they were met by a man she subsequently identified as Jack Ruby. She did not know who Ruby was, and only learned of his identity after Ruby shot Oswald and appeared on television. Ruby spoke only with Sturgis in the parking lot of the motel. Ruby apparently objected to having a woman in the group, and Sturgis sent Lorenz back to Miami on an airplane.

Lorenz also testified that after Watergate she was visited by an FBI case agent who showed her a newspaper containing photos of Frank Sturgis and E. Howard Hunt. She identified Sturgis using the name by which she had known him, Frank Fiorini, and identified Hunt as "Eduardo", who she had met several times, and who had supplied Operation 40 figures with money. She identified Hunt and Sturgis as friends.

During her testimony Lorenz was threatened with federal perjury charges when it was pointed out to her that Lee Harvey Oswald was in the Soviet Union at the time she said she met him at the Florida Everglades training camp, and that Oswald was working a regular job at the Dallas School Book Depository at the time she said he was engaged in Operation 40 activities in Miami, and then traveled from Miami to Dallas. Even in the face of threatened federal perjury charges Lorenz steadfastly insisted that the Oswald she knew in Florida was the same Oswald that she saw on television after the assassination.

In subsequent testimony, Frank Sturgis vigorously denied Lorenz' allegations. The House Select Committee found Lorenz' testimony to be unreliable, based largely on the impossibility of her having met and observed Oswald in the stated time frame. The House Select Committee failed to consider the possibility that Lorenz had not only observed an Oswald double, but that the double was impersonating Oswald as early as 1960. [14]

It has been established that after Oswald defected to the Soviet Union, the FBI became concerned that someone was impersonating him. In June 1960 J. Edgar Hoover sent the State Department a memorandum stating: "Since there is a possibility that an imposter is using Oswald's birth certificate, any current information the Department of State may have concerning subject will be appreciated."[15] Lorenz' adamant insistence in the face of threatened perjury charges that she knew and traveled with "Lee Harvey Oswald" parallels Deputy Sheriff Roger Craig's equally strenuous insistence that he saw Lee Harvey Oswald exit the Texas School Book Depository fifteen minutes after the assassination and loudly hail a station wagon resembling the one owned by Ruth Paine. Both episodes suggest the presence of an Oswald lookalike double, who many believe to be an individual named William Seymour.

The fact that Lorenz' "Lee Harvey Oswald" was a trained Operation 40 assassin who traveled to Dallas adds to the possibility that an Oswald double could have been present in the Texas School Book Depository and fired upon the President.

The House Select Committee chose not to believe Marita Lorenz' allegations concerning Lee Harvey Oswald and Operation 40. However, E. Howard Hunt's deathbed confession that the assassination was originally scheduled for Miami, then changed to Dallas, breathes new life into Lorenz' story of a sudden trip to Dallas undertaken by Operation 40 personnel. Lorenz made the allegations in 1978, long before E. Howard Hunt's deathbed confession became known.

President Kennedy visited Miami on Monday, November 18, 1963, four days before his murder.

CHAPTER 9

PERMINDEX, THE ASSASSINATION CORPORATION

Jim Garrison's investigation of Clay Shaw eventually traced Shaw's activities back to his work as a director of Permindex, an international corporation that was located in Geneva, Switzerland. The investigation also established that Major Louis Mortimer Bloomfield, a former agent for the Office of Strategic Services (OSS), predecessor of the CIA, was a major shareholder in Permindex and its sister organization in Rome, the Centro Mondiale Commerciale (World Trade Center). As part of his service with the OSS, Bloomfield worked for the FBI's Division Five counter-intelligence bureau, and became quite close to FBI Director J. Edgar Hoover.[1] The Italian Press eventually unmasked the Centro Mondiale Commerciale as "a creature of the CIA…set up as a cover for the transfer of CIA…funds in Italy for illegal political-espionage activities".[2]

Permindex was the primary focus of a document that surfaced anonymously among assassination researchers in 1970. That document was called the "Torbitt Document", after the author's *nom de plume*, William Torbitt. While the document makes some wild allegations, it presents a very clear, very detailed, very comprehensive picture of the assassination, as told by its anonymous author. It identifies and ties together many specific names, dates, and events associated with the assassination and it is clear that the author has a deeply ingrained insider's knowledge of events leading up to, during, and after the assassination. Many of the individuals discussed in Torbitt otherwise appear in the assassination investigation and documentation for no apparent reason, and Torbitt explains their presence.

Torbitt was presented to the public in 1996 in a book entitled *NASA, Nazis and JFK: The Torbitt Document and the JFK Assassination*.[3] It is unfortunate that the authors chose to sensationalize Torbitt by associating it with NASA and the Nazis. While remnants of Hitler's intelligence apparatus did play a role in the founding of Permindex, the Torbitt account does not assign a substantial role to either NASA nor former Nazis in the plot to kill the President.*

It is not clear to this day who Torbitt is. In *NASA, Nazis and JFK* it is claimed that the author is a Texas lawyer with experience in investigations and prosecutions of gambling syndicates and the Mafia. The information in Torbitt was allegedly contained in a working paper that Torbitt received from two agents within the Customs Department and Narcotics Bureau.[4] Many believe that Torbitt was Texas lawyer David Copeland, who was intimately familiar with the Johnson political machine in Texas. [5]

The document, however, could easily have been composed by more than one author, given the specificity and detail of insider knowledge required in different fields, including the Garrison investigation, as well as the inner workings of the CIA and Division Five, the counter-espionage section of the FBI.

The New Orleans District Attorney files are cited extensively in Torbitt. Jim Garrison or an office colleague could have been Torbitt, or one of several authors of Torbitt. However, since Garrison's files were allegedly stolen by CIA operative William Wood, aka "Bill Boxley", the circle of potential authors extends well beyond the District Attorney's office.[6] Other possibilities include manufacture by the CIA to deflect mounting blame from itself, or even the Soviet KGB, to emphasize the role of anti-Soviet Fascists in the operation that took the President's life.

In Torbitt the roles of the CIA and FBI relative to Permindex are reversed. According to Torbitt, the CIA played a minimal role, and J. Edgar Hoover and the FBI largely controlled Permindex' activities. Torbitt bluntly tells the reader that "The killing of President Kennedy was planned and supervised by Division Five of the Federal Bureau of Investigation, a relatively small department within the FBI whose usual duties are espionage and counter-espionage activities". [7]

Division Five had its origins in the General Intelligence Division of the

---

* It should be noted, however, that within weeks of the assassination many of Oswald's former co-workers at the Reilly Coffee Company went to work for NASA and related contractors.

Department of Justice in 1919. When J. Edgar Hoover became the FBI's first director in 1924, he incorporated Division Five into the FBI for espionage and counter-espionage work, an administrative move that was eventually formalized by President Roosevelt in 1936. [8]

In the early 1930s J. Edgar Hoover organized the police force of the Tennessee Valley Authority (TVA), a New Deal project designed to dam and create electricity along the Tennessee River. The TVA was one of the first federal agencies to have its own police force, and it covered the area from Knoxville, Tennessee to Huntsville, Alabama, and into Kentucky. The force grew to cover the Atomic Energy Commission,* creating an interface with the Army intelligence service, and eventually it became a sprawling government entity known as the Defense Industrial Security Command (DISC). [9]

The Defense Industrial Security Command was supervised by Division Five of the FBI until 1961, when control of DISC became shared with the newly created Defense Intelligence Agency (DIA). The head of the DIA was Lieutenant General Joseph Carroll, a former Assistant Director of the FBI, and personnel within the DIA were subject to assignment in DISC. The activities of DISC were largely kept secret, but it became a sprawling bureaucracy whose primary mission was to provide security services to NASA, the Atomic Energy Commission, the U.S. Information Agency, and the Pentagon, as well as all arms and equipment manufacturers contracting with those agencies. [10]

According to Torbitt DISC controlled Permindex, which was used to finance, direct, and coordinate five distinct entities:

1. The Solidarists: an anti-Soviet organization of White Russians and similarly minded individuals headed by Ferenc Nagy, former premier of Hungary, and Jean de Menil, a Russian exile who had fled to France, married into the Schlumberger family, and became Chairman of the Board of the Schlumberger Corporation. De Menil was a close friend and supporter of Lyndon Johnson for over thirty years.

---

* Oak Ridge, Tennessee was one of the primary research and development sites for the creation of atomic weapons for the Manhattan Project during World War II.

2. The American Council of Christian Churches: an intelligence and espionage organization created by J. Edgar Hoover in 1941, with headquarters in New York City. Its purpose was to provide an umbrella organization for religious groups that were largely ignorant of its real mission, which was to place agents posing as ministers and missionaries throughout North and South America. The organization was headed by H.L. Hunt of Dallas, Texas.*

3. The Free Cuba Committee: a Cuban exile group headed by Carlos Prio Socarras, the former President of Cuba.**

4. The Syndicate: an organization of gamblers headed by Clifford Jones, former Lieutenant Governor of Nevada, and Bobby Baker, a close associate of Lyndon Johnson. This group was closely affiliated with the Bonanno crime family.

5. The Security Division of NASA: the headquarters for this group was the Defense Industrial Security Group at the Muscle Shoals Redstone Arsenal, Alabama, and Columbus, Ohio facilities. The division was headed by former Nazi rocket scientist Werner von Braun. [12]

DISC was organized by J. Edgar Hoover. Hoover's assistant, William Sullivan, was head of Division Five, and thus in direct control of DISC.*** Torbitt states that Clay Shaw, David Ferrie, Jack Ruby, Lee Harvey Oswald, and Guy Banister were DISC agents who were supervised directly by

---

* The West Coast representative of the American Council of Christian Churches, E.E. Bradley, was indicted by a New Orleans Grand Jury for complicity in the assassination of President Kennedy.
** Prio Socarras was shot to death before the House Select Committee on Assassinations could speak with him. [11]
*** In 1977 Sullivan was shot to death before he could speak to the House Select Committee on Assassinations, in what was alleged to have been a hunting accident. He once told reporter Robert Novak that "Someday, you will read that I have been killed in an accident, but don't believe it, I've been murdered." [13] Sullivan's obituary states that his career with the FBI began in the early days of World War II, when Hoover sent him on an undercover intelligence assignment in Europe. [14]

Permindex' L.M. Bloomfield in Montreal. Bloomfield held fifty percent of the shares in Permindex and was a longtime friend and confidant of J. Edgar Hoover, dating back to Bloomfield's days in the Office of Strategic Services. According to Torbitt, Bloomfield was the coordinator of all plans for the assassination, answering only to J. Edgar Hoover and Lyndon Johnson. [15]

The stated purpose of Permindex was to facilitate international trade, but according to Torbitt its actual mission was to:

1. Fund and direct assassinations of European, Mid-East and world leaders deemed threats to the Western World and to the petroleum interests of its backers.

2. To furnish couriers, agents, and management for the transporting, depositing, and rechanneling of funds through Swiss banks for Las Vegas, Miami, Havana, and international gambling syndicates.

3. To coordinate the espionage activities of the Solidarists and Division Five with groups sympathetic to their objectives, and to channel funds and arms to those groups to achieve their objectives.

4. To acquire, build, and operate hotels and casinos in Italy, the Caribbean, and other tourist areas. [16]

In addition to the murder of President Kennedy, Torbitt ties Permindex to several other assassinations. In the early 1960s France was paralyzed by the attempt of Algeria to free itself from French colonial rule. French President Charles de Gaulle favored decolonization, but was opposed by a group of right wing generals who wanted to keep Algeria as a French colony.

In 1962 French Colonel Bastien Thiry commanded a group of assassins who fired on de Gaulle's limousine in the suburbs of Paris. The attempt was unsuccessful, and de Gaulle escaped unscathed. Thiry was arrested, tried, and executed for the attempt on de Gaulle's life. French intelligence eventually traced funding for the assassination to Permindex in Switzerland, then into NATO headquarters in Brussels, Belgium. Enraged, de Gaulle pulled France out of NATO. The story eventually found its way onto the pages of prominent French newspapers such as *Le Monde* and *L'Express*. [17]

Guy Banister had been head of the FBI's Chicago office until 1955, when Hoover shifted him to contract work on behalf of Division Five, first within the New Orleans Police Department, then as a private detective. Banister sent Maurice Gatlin, General Counsel to the Anti-Communist League of the Caribbean, from New Orleans to Paris with $100,000 in cash for the planners of the de Gaulle assassination. In 1964 Gatlin died from a mysterious fall in the middle of the night from the El Panama Hotel in Panama.[18] Banister also died in 1964.

Torbitt believes that Hoover, Bloomfield, and Permindex also planned and executed the assassinations of Robert Kennedy and Martin Luther King. He notes that James Earl Ray, the accused and convicted assassin of Martin Luther King, was a frequent visitor to the New Orleans International Trade Mart, run by Clay Shaw. [19]

Torbitt describes how many of the interlocking relationships that surfaced in the Kennedy assassination predate Castro's revolution and go back to the days of Joseph McCarthy's anti-Communist crusade in the Senate.

Morris Dalitz was a prominent Cleveland, Ohio mobster who had been a business partner of the Bonanno crime family. He eventually came to control the infamous Stardust Hotel in Las Vegas. Dalitz, Roy Cohn (McCarthy's Senate legal counsel), H.L. Hunt, and J. Edgar Hoover all worked together in anti-Communist activities during the McCarthy years in the early 1950s. [20-22]

In 1969 author Ed Reid published a book entitled *The Grim Reapers* that included a photo of Lyndon Johnson at the Stardust Hotel when Johnson and Bobby Baker met with Dalitz prior to the assassination. Johnson and Dalitz were photographed together a number of times during this meeting, which included Johnson, Baker, Dalitz, Roy Cohn, and Clifford Jones. [23, 24]

There were also connections between Hoover's intelligence empire and organized crime through legitimate business enterprises. Both Joe Bonanno and Roy Cohn were closely associated with Lionel, a munitions manufacturing corporation, and as such, would have been subject to scrutiny by DISC.[25] Senate investigations in the 1960s turned up hidden connections between Medico Industries, a Pentagon contractor, and Sicilian-born Russell Bufalino, described as "one of the most ruthless and powerful leaders of the Mafia in the United States".[26] Until 1959 Hoover steadfastly denied the existence of the Mafia. The Mafia was also connected to Permindex through Rome's Centro Mondiale Commerciale and its Italian Mafia director, Gutierez di Spadafora. [27, 28]

Torbitt asserts that Lee Harvey Oswald was recruited for Division Five work by David Ferrie in 1956 before Oswald joined the Marines. He was paid through an account in the Department of Immigration and Naturalization, a method that Hoover used to pay covert agents. The address of the Dallas office of the Department of Immigration and Naturalization was found in Oswald's notebook. This gave rise to allegations that were forwarded to the Warren Commission by Dallas District Attorney Henry Wade and Texas Attorney General Waggoner Carr that Oswald was being paid $200 per month by the FBI using informant number S-172. [29]

Instead of examining the matter, the Commission reflexly regarded the information as a false rumor that had to be suppressed.

The Warren Commission went to great lengths to tell America that Lee Harvey Oswald had absolutely nothing to do with the individual sitting next to him on his bus trip to Mexico City prior to the assassination:

"The investigation of the Commission has produced considerable testimonial and documentary evidence establishing the precise time of Oswald's journey, his means of transportation, the hotel at which he stayed in Mexico City, and a restaurant at which he often ate. All known persons whom Oswald may have met while in Mexico, including passengers on the buses he rode, and the employees and guests of the hotel where he stayed, were interviewed. No credible witness has been located who saw Oswald with any unidentified person while in Mexico City; to the contrary, he was observed traveling alone to and from Mexico City, at his hotel, and at the nearby restaurant where he frequently ate. A hotel guest stated that on one occasion he sat down at a table with Oswald at the restaurant because no empty table was available, but that neither spoke to the other because of the language barrier. Two Australian girls who saw Oswald on the bus to Mexico City relate that he occupied a seat next to a man who has been identified as Albert Osborne, an elderly itinerant preacher. Osborne denies that Oswald was beside him on the bus. To the other passengers on the bus it appeared that Osborne and Oswald had not previously met, and extensive investigation of Osborne has revealed no further contact between him and Oswald. Osborne's responses to federal investigators on matters unrelated to Oswald have proved inconsistent and unreliable, and, therefore, based on the contrary evidence and Osborne's lack of reliability, the

Commission has attached no credence to his denial that Oswald was beside him on the bus. Investigation of his background and activities, however, disclose no basis for suspecting him of any involvement in the assassination." [30]

When the FBI first interviewed the man who had been sitting next to Oswald on the bus, he stated that his name was John Howard Bowen. During a subsequent interview he recanted, and said that his name was actually Albert Alexander Osborne. [31]

According to Torbitt, Albert Alexander Osborne, alias John Howard Bowen, was a charter member of the American Council of Christian Churches. He worked for Division Five of the FBI maintaining a stable of 25 – 30 professional rifleman in Mexico who were used for political killings all over the world for 25 years. The existence of such a group came to light during an investigation by the Texas Attorney General's office into a botched political assassination involving a District Judge in Alice, Texas. When not posing as missionaries in Mexico, Osborne and his charges were based at Clint Murchison's Texas ranch. [32]

Clint Murchison's largesse also extended to J. Edgar Hoover himself. Hoover was a frequent visitor to the Del Charro Hotel, adjacent to Murchison's horseracing track at La Jolla, California, where he charged over $40,000 of his personal bills to Murchison's Delhi-Taylor Oil Company. From 1953 to 1963 Hoover and Murchison met frequently at Del Charro with John Connally, Carlos Marcello, Joe Bonanno, and other Mafia figures. [33]

To achieve its goals, Permindex set up a subsidiary in the U.S. called Double-Chek. One of the employees of Double-Chek was William Seymour, said to be an exact double of Lee Harvey Oswald, differing only in that he maintained an unkempt appearance, unlike Oswald, who was usually clean shaven and well groomed. Seymour was assigned the alias Leon Oswald, and is thought to have made appearances in Miami, New Orleans, and Dallas masquerading as Oswald. Many believe that Seymour was the individual observed by Deputy Sheriff Roger Craig exiting the School Book Depository fifteen minutes after the assassination and loudly hailing a Nash Rambler station wagon on Elm Street. [34]

Torbitt also takes aim at the large number of "sex deviates" in and around the assassination:

167

"L.M. Bloomfield, a Montreal, Canada lawyer bearing the reputation as a sex deviate, the direct supervisor of all contractual agents with J. Edgar Hoover's Division Five, was the top coordinator for the network planning the execution..." [35]

"Clay Shaw and Walter Jenkins, only two of the large number of sex deviates at command and lower level of the cabal, were together almost constantly, pushing L.B.J. during the 1960 Democratic Convention in Los Angeles according to delegates presented there..." [36]

Despite the fact that it is well sourced, the Torbitt document must, of necessity, be regarded with some degree of skepticism due to its murky origins. It is, however, no accident that Permindex' involvement in the Kennedy assassination was eventually uncovered and documented.

Jim Garrison unmasked Clay Shaw because Shaw contacted New Orleans attorney Dean Andrews to represent Oswald right after the assassination. Clay Shaw had previously referred Oswald to Andrews. Clay Shaw was a director of Permindex. Permindex was involved in assassination attempts on French President Charles de Gaulle. The path from Assassination, Inc. runs straight through Clay Shaw to Lee Harvey Oswald. The connections are all very clear and all very well documented. [37]

Political scientist Jerome Corsi explored the origins of Permindex in his recent book, *Who Really Killed Kennedy?* In the years before World War II, the grandfathers of Allen Dulles, John Foster Dulles and President George H.W. Bush worked to finance the rise of Adolf Hitler in Germany. In the 1920s the Bush and Dulles families became involved with the Harriman investment banking empire, and in particular, with large sums of Nazi-related money that were transferred into the coffers of the Union Banking Corporation. The bank was closed after Germany declared war on the United States.

In the 1920s both Allen Dulles and John Foster Dulles joined the prestigious New York law firm of Sullivan and Cromwell. Sullivan and Cromwell did work for the German chemical giant I.G. Farben, manufacturer of Zyklon-B, the gas used to exterminate inmates in concentration camps. John Foster Dulles would sign I.G. Farben correspondence with "Heil Hitler".

After Hitler's rise to power, Allen Dulles was a director of the New York branch of the J. Henry Schroeder Bank, ultimately becoming Schroeder Bank's general counsel. The Schroeder family in Germany included Baron Kurt von Schroeder, who was a special agent for Heinrich Himmler, head of the Gestapo secret police and the dreaded SS (Schutzstaffel).

At the end of World War II Allen Dulles was chief of the Berlin office of the Office of Strategic Services. He secured the release of the director of Nazi intelligence, Reinhard Gehlen, from a prison camp and set in motion a strategy of deploying former Nazi intelligence assets to the advantage of the United States. Gehlen eventually became the intelligence chief for the Federal Republic of West Germany.

After the war Germany was transformed into a Cold War ally against the threat of Soviet expansionism, and individuals and firms with prewar financial experience in Germany found themselves possessing a unique kind of information and expertise that made them invaluable to the American intelligence community.

In the 1950s and 60s the J. Henry Schroeder Banking Corporation and Schroeder Trust became depositories for CIA money. When Allen Dulles was head of the CIA the secret depository amounted to fifty million dollars, personally controlled by Dulles. In 1956 the J. Henry Schroeder Banking Corporation financed the opening of Permindex, later to come under the glare of the media spotlight for having financed assassination attempts on Charles de Gaulle, and for potential involvement in the assassination of President Kennedy. [38]

CHAPTER 10

J. EDGAR HOOVER, THE TWISTED MAN

It is unlikely that there will ever be a prominent figure in the federal government quite like J. Edgar Hoover.

His twisted life as a closet homosexual and transvestite, his immense hypocrisy of accusing others of "sexual deviancy", his creation of a secret police force designed to spy on the most intimate aspects of American life, his alliances with significant crime figures, and his constant use of blackmail to intimidate presidents and prominent politicians all register in stark contrast to his public persona as a man of morals, creator of an efficient and professional federal police force, and effective leader of an America free from Communist tyranny and subversion. [1]

All suggest the profile of a thoroughly deranged man who would do anything to acquire and maintain power over the American people.

J. Edgar Hoover was appointed the first Director of the FBI in 1924 by Attorney General Harlan Fiske Stone as part of a reorganization of the Bureau of Investigation within the Department of Justice. In the 1920s and 30s Hoover achieved a number of successes, including the establishment of a forensics laboratory, a national training academy, and the apprehension of notorious bank robbers. He elevated the status of the Bureau in the public eye by establishing and promoting a national bulletin called "Fugitives Wanted by Police", forerunner of today's "Ten Most Wanted List". Hoover created a centralized fingerprint registry, although his dream of "universal fingerprinting" - the fingerprinting of all U.S. citizens – never came to fruition. [2]

In running the Bureau, Hoover acquired a reputation as a tyrannical despot. Hoover intervened in all aspects of agents' lives. Unmarried agents were to forego having sex. He intervened in marriages that did not meet his approval, and kept tabs on agents' extramarital affairs. Hoover criticized one agent in front of his colleagues for possessing a copy of *Playboy*, publicly denouncing those who read such magazines as "moral degenerates". [3]

Hoover routinely sent his "goon squads" to Bureau offices to detect and punish even the slightest transgressions. Agents who displeased him were either fired outright, or given a series of transfers to remote Bureau locations designed to encourage them to quit. [4]

Hoover obtained a charter for the Bureau's own Masonic lodge. Membership was voluntary, but a prerequisite for advancement. Hoover himself eventually rose to the position of 33rd degree Mason, the highest rank possible. In hiring new agents, Hoover felt that the ideal candidate included membership in the Masons, and as a result, few Catholics rose to top positions within the Bureau for many years. [5,6]

Richard Nixon was well aware of how Hoover's status in Washington complicated Nixon's political calculus:

Richard Nixon: For a lot of reasons he oughta resign...He should get the hell out of there...Now it may be, which I kind of doubt... maybe I could just call him and talk him into resigning...There are some problems...If he does go he's got to go of his own volition... that's why we're in a hell of a problem...I think he'll stay until he's a hundred years old.

John Mitchell: He'll stay until he's buried there. Immortality…

Richard Nixon: I think we've got to avoid the situation where he can leave with a blast…We may have on our hands here a man who will pull down the temple with him, including me…It's going to be a problem. [7]

Agents would privately deride Hoover as "Kid Napoleon", a reference, in part, to his short stature. Hoover stood approximately 5' 7", and attempted to disguise his height through various means. Hoover's desk and chair were installed on a platform, and visitors would sit on a low couch, such that Hoover would be looking down at them. Hoover's shoes were custom built to give him the appearance of being taller. [8]

Hoover's undertaker once remarked that Hoover's house "was like a museum. Like a shrine the man had made to himself. He must've had some ego. The picture of him at the top of the stairs was almost like the one of Napoleon with the hand inside of the jacket." Another colleague observed several statues that were "busts, like Roman busts of Caesar, but of J. Edgar Hoover". [9]

Not all of the agents were targets of Hoover's tyranny. Clyde Tolson was hired by the Bureau in 1928, and within three years Hoover had promoted him to Assistant Director, Hoover's second in command. Like Hoover, Tolson was homosexual, and he soon became Hoover's constant companion. Tolson took great pleasure in acting as Hoover's administrative hatchet man within the Bureau. [10] *

Hoover's secret life was hardly a secret amongst the well informed, including the Mafia. Meyer Lansky and his associate Lewis Rosensteil were both well aware of Hoover's proclivities. Rosensteil's wife described seeing Hoover dressed up as a woman:

> "He was wearing a fluffy black dress, very fluffy, with flounces, and lace stockings and high heels, and a black curly wig. He had makeup on, and false eyelashes. It was a very short skirt, and he was sitting there in the living room of the suite with his legs crossed. Roy (Cohn) introduced him to me as 'Mary'...It was obvious he wasn't a woman, you could see where he shaved. It was Hoover. You've never seen anything like it. I couldn't believe it, that I should see the head of the FBI dressed as a woman...The next thing, a couple of boys come in, young blond boys. I'd say about eighteen or nineteen...And they go into the bedroom, and Hoover takes off his lace dress and pants, and under the dress he was wearing a little, short garter belt. He lies on the double bed, and the two boys work on him with their hands. One of them wore rubber gloves..." [12]

---

* In his book *The Bureau* William Sullivan relates a story about Tolson: "A story that may or not be true went the rounds of the bureau that Tolson came into work one day complaining to Hoover that he was depressed. To cheer him up, Hoover gave Tolson a list of FBI supervisors. 'Pick out one you don't like and fire him,' the director said, 'then you'll feel better.'...Tolson then smiled at Hoover and asked, 'With prejudice?'." [11]

A year later she and Rosensteil again visited the Plaza, and Cohn introduced them to Hoover in drag:

"He had a red dress on, and a black feather boa around his neck... After about half an hour some boys came, like before. This time they're dressed in leather. And Hoover had a Bible. He wanted one of the boys to read from the Bible. And he read, I forgot which passage, and the other boy played with him, wearing the rubber gloves. And then Hoover grabbed the Bible, threw it down and told the second boy to join in the sex." [13]

The Mafia ultimately used Hoover's indiscretions to carve out a symbiotic relationship with him, the Mafia benefiting from willful inattention to their misdeeds and Hoover benefiting from his continued status as a pillar of virtue and paragon of moral society. The Mafia sweetened the pot by throwing in tips on fixed horseraces that Hoover could cash in on, especially when they socialized together at Clint Murchison's Del Mar racetrack. [14]

The Master of Ceremonies for Hoover's transvestite *soirées* was lawyer Roy Cohn, who had become famous during the 1950s as legal counsel to Senator Joseph McCarthy's hearings into Communist subversion. The hearings came at a time of mounting military and geopolitical tensions between the Unites States and its Communist foes, including, in particular, the Soviet Union.*

McCarthy was first elected to the Senate from Wisconsin in 1946. By 1950 he had achieved fame by charging that the State Department was full of Communists, and he instigated a nationwide crusade against the Red Menace. Numerous hearings were held in which accusations of support

---

* During World War II the United States and Soviet Union were allies of convenience against a common enemy, Nazi Germany. After much of eastern Europe was overrun by the Soviet Union at the end of the war, the diplomatic posture of the two countries changed dramatically, and the Cold War ensued. In the U.S. anti-Communist sentiment soared with the conviction of Julius and Ethel Rosenberg for atomic spying, the explosion of the Soviet Union's first atomic bomb, and the Communist takeover of mainland China.

for Communism were leveled, but rarely proven. Many were blacklisted from employment or otherwise publicly condemned on the word of J. Edgar Hoover that they were disloyal to the United States. At the same time Hoover started a similar campaign against homosexuals, especially those in government, that came to be known as the Lavender Scare. After Communists, homosexuals in government became one of McCarthy's primary targets.

In the midst of McCarthy's witch hunt an article appeared on the October 25, 1952 pages of the Las Vegas Sun accusing McCarthy himself of homosexuality. Editor Hank Greenspun wrote a front page editorial in response to McCarthy's having called him an "Ex-Communist" at a speech in Nevada.

Greenspun catalogued a number of McCarthy associates who had been publicly exposed as gay, going so far as to detail McCarthy's bedroom stay at a state convention with William McMahon, a former official of the Milwaukee County Young Republicans. Greenspun stated that it was "common talk among homosexuals in Milwaukee who rendezvous at the White Horse Inn that Sen. Joe McCarthy has often engaged in homosexual activities."

Greenspun also highlighted McCarthy's hypocrisy of accusing the State Department of being "honeycombed" with homosexuals in light of his own conduct. McCarthy denied the allegations and soon afterward married his secretary and adopted a daughter.

If rumors of McCarthy's homosexuality were true, it would appear then that McCarthyism itself was presided over by a *troika* of homosexuals – Joseph McCarthy, Roy Cohn,* and J. Edgar Hoover - who commandeered the machinery of media and government to make wild accusations and ruin reputations based on whispers, whim, and puffed up allegations with little or no merit. As a result of McCarthyism, Hoover's media machine ensured that he would become one of the most influential and respected men in the United States. In the 1950s and early 60s many considered his pronouncements to be godlike.

---

* McCarthy was accused of making allegations that the U.S. Army harbored Communists because the Army would not grant special treatment to Cohn's homosexual boyfriend, David Schine. Cohn always denied that he was gay, but he eventually died of AIDS in 1986.

One of Hoover's major achievements at the Bureau was to create a centralized filing system that allowed for the rapid indexing and retrieval of agent's reports. This included an "Obscene File", as well as a "Sex Deviate" card file that was used to smear various politicians, as well as provide information concerning suitability for employment in the federal civil service. [15] *

This tactic was used to accumulate gossip and innuendo about the 1952 and 1956 Democrat candidate for President, Adlai Stevenson, who was featured in several reports:

Informal memo, FBI Assistant Director D. Milton Ladd to FBI Director, June 24, 1952:

Pursuant to your request, there is attached hereto a blind memorandum concerning Governor Stevenson, who, it has been alleged, is a known homosexual...

An official of the City of New York ascertained from an individual, as well as from a public official, both from the State of Illinois, that Governor Adlai Ewing Stevenson was one of the best-known homosexuals in the State of Illinois. Stevenson was allegedly well-known as "Adeline." Because of Stevenson's being a homosexual, it was the opinion of the individuals who made this statement that he would not run for President in 1952. [17]

Informal Memo, FBI Supervisor Milton Jones to FBI Assistant Director Louis Nichols, July 24, 1952:

...In April, 1952, the New York Office received confidential information from a detective of the New York District Attorney's office to the effect that Adlai Stevenson and David B. Owen, President, Bradley University, Peoria, Illinois, were two officials in Illinois who caused a great deal of trouble to law enforcement

---

* When the FBI destroyed the Sexual Deviates Indexes and Files in 1977, they numbered over 300,000 pages. [16]

officers.

The detective had gone to Peoria to bring back basketball players who had been indicted in New York. The basketball players told the detective that the two best-known homo-sexuals in Illinois were Owen and Stevenson. According to the report, Stevenson was known as "Adeline." [18]

Informal memo, FBI Assistant Director D. Milton Ladd to FBI Director, August 15, 1952:

[Assistant SAC Washington] Fletcher...[reported having learned] that there was some high official alleged to be spreading word that [Adlai] Stevenson was a "queer"; that the FBI had a file on him. Further that the Democratic National Committee was very angry about the situation...[19]

In a twist of irony, while Hoover was using the Sex Deviate card file to accumulate a mountain of dirt on homosexuals in America, FBI agents were routinely sent out to interview and intimidate anyone found to have expressed the opinion that Hoover was homosexual, "queer", or a "sissy". [20]

Because the records in the centralized filing system were subject to court-ordered or congressional access, Hoover devised procedures to maintain sensitive materials outside the reach of external scrutiny: first, certain types of information were maintained in files located in the Director's office, and second, he created a reporting procedure called "personal and confidential" letters, in which communications from field office heads or special agents in charge could be routed around the Bureau's indexed central records system. [21]

In this manner the Bureau's illegal investigative techniques – black-bag jobs, wiretaps, bugs, and especially the intimate bedroom spying that served as Hoover's blackmail ammunition - could escape detection. It also allowed Hoover to accumulate and maintain a massive collection of all manner of pornography in his office. Hoover even installed a special movie room to view these materials. [22]

Hoover's files demonstrate his early fascination with Kennedy's sex life. Inga Arvad was a columnist for the Washington Times-Herald. She was a former Miss Denmark who was suspected of having pro-Nazi leanings. An FBI investigation uncovered no evidence of espionage, but Hoover nonetheless went ahead and bugged her hotel room: [23]

Personal and Confidential Report of Special Agent Savannah Office to Washington Office, February 9, 1942. Synopsis of facts:

Surveillance maintained upon [Arvad] from the time of her arrival in Charleston, S.C. at 8:20 A.M. on 2-6-42 until her departure therefrom on 2-9-42 at 1:09 A.M. to return to Washington, D.C. While there, John Kennedy, Ensign U.S. Navy, spent each night with subject in her hotel room at the Fort Sumter Hotel, engaging in sexual intercourse on numerous occasions...Only information gained by [Arvad] of possible espionage value, fact that Kennedy proceeding to Norfolk, Va. soon for training, fire control work, also serious illness of Harry Hopkins, Presidential Advisor...

At Charleston, South Carolina:

At 8:20 A.M. on February 6, 1942, [Arvad] arrived at the Union Station in Charleston, South Carolina, where she was met by John Kennedy...Mrs. Fejos registered at the Fort Sumter Hotel approximately at 8:55 A.M., on the same date as her arrival, using the name Barbara White. A twenty-four hour surveillance was maintained from that point on until the subject departed from Charleston...

From a strongly confidential source [a bug in their hotel room], a great deal of the conversation which passed between [Arvad] and Kennedy in the hotel room was obtained. The majority of this conversation was of little interest in this particular case.

Shortly prior to subject's departure on the evening of February 8, Kennedy made out a check payable to [Arvad] in an amount which could not be ascertained. After he made out this check, he asked [Arvad] if it were sufficient, to which she replied in the affirmative.

From this same [microphone installation] it was determined that Kennedy and Mrs. Fejos engaged in sexual intercourse on a number of occasions from February 6, 1942, until February 9, 1942. Kennedy spent the nights of February 6, 7, and 8th in the subject's hotel room, staying all night there after she had left for Washington, D.C., as set out above.

The only information pertaining to Kennedy's official movements that was obtained from their conversation was the fact that he expected to go to Norfolk, Virginia within the next four to five days for a period of three weeks to study fire control. She did not press him further as to his future plans, or for any information concerning the movements of any vessels belonging to the United States Navy. As to her movements, she stated that she was going to return to Washington to go back to work and was seriously considering going to Reno to get a divorce from her present husband and marry Kennedy. [24]

At the time of Kennedy's assassination Hoover had been close friends with Lyndon Johnson for many years. Hoover had known Johnson since the 1930s, and since the 1940s he was a close neighbor, living only three houses away. Hoover was a regular visitor to the Johnson household, and even filled in as a baby sitter for Johnson's daughters. Johnson, by then acknowledged as one of the most corrupt politicians in Washington, saw the obvious value in cultivating Hoover as a friend and ally. According to William Sullivan, Hoover and Johnson were frequent dinner guests at each others homes.[25] Hoover campaigned on behalf of Johnson for President in 1960, unheard of behavior for a police official.

When Johnson failed to get the nomination, Hoover provided the blackmail leverage to force Johnson onto the ticket.[26] During the election, Hoover ordered the bugging of the plane of Kennedy's opponent.

There are many potential scenarios linking Hoover to the assassination. These run the gamut from his playing an active role in the planning and execution of Kennedy's murder via Division Five and Permindex, to simply looking the other way in the face of Mafia plots or the danger posed by an alleged Communist fanatic like Oswald, to actively obfuscating the investigation after the fact.

178

J. EDGAR HOOVER

In assessing Hoover's role in the assassination it must be kept in mind that he was present in Dallas, along with Lyndon Johnson and Richard Nixon, at a party thrown by Clint Murchison the night before the assassination. In fact, the party was thrown in Hoover's honor.

Richard Case Nagell served as a U.S. Military Intelligence Officer from 1955 to 1959, and was employed by the CIA as a contract agent from 1962 to 1963. His assignment for the CIA was to carefully monitor Lee Harvey Oswald in the months prior to the assassination.* By late in the summer of 1963 he had become aware of a large and well organized assassination plot involving Oswald. Nagell determined that Guy Banister, Clay Shaw, and David Ferrie were manipulating Oswald prior to the assassination. [29]

In September 1963 Nagell sent a registered letter to J. Edgar Hoover warning him of the plot to assassinate the President, specifically naming Oswald as a key figure. Nagell listed pertinent facts about Oswald, including his physical description, known aliases, and his residential address. Nagell then proceeded to shoot up a federally insured bank in El Paso and directed the investigating FBI agents to examine the intelligence materials in the trunk of his car. At a preliminary hearing before the assassination Nagell told the original arresting policeman that he had acted because he didn't want "to be in Dallas", to which the officer replied "What do you mean by that?". Nagell's response was "You'll see soon enough", which the officer later came to understand as foretelling the assassination.**

---

* Author Dick Russell eventually received a Military Intelligence file confirming Nagell's assertions that he had been working for the CIA in the months prior to the assassination, and that he had been assigned to monitor Oswald. [27] The Warren Commission attempted to minimize the level of interaction between the federal government and Oswald, but it is clear that the federal government had Oswald under close surveillance in the weeks immediately preceding the assassination. In an article published in the New York Times three days after the assassination, William Kline, the assistant U.S. Customs agent in charge of the investigative service in Laredo, Texas, stated that "Oswald's movements were watched at the request of a federal agency in Washington", who he declined to name. [28]

** Nagell was found dead one day after the JFK Assassination Records Review Board sent him a letter notifying him that he was to testify before the Board. His death was attributed to a heart attack, although he had no

179

Nagell's warning letter and treasure trove of intelligence documentation were ignored by Hoover and the FBI.[30] The key question of course is why would Hoover's fanatically anti-Communist FBI ignore such assertions about an apparent Communist sympathizer like Oswald?

In 1962 FBI agent M. Wesley Swearington received information from a Cuban exile informant that plans were being made to kill President Kennedy. The plot originated with those training to kill Castro, and had a similar methodology, namely a designated "patsy" would fire the first shot and then be killed and subsequently blamed for the assassination. CIA agent William Harvey was identified as part of the plot, as well as Guy Banister, who was setting up the unidentified "patsy", said to have been a real "nutcase". Swearington filed a report, which was ignored, and his reward was a prompt transfer to Paintsville, Kentucky. [31]

By many accounts Hoover had an intense hatred of both Jack and Robert Kennedy. He resented President Kennedy's youthfulness and his liberal legislative agenda, particularly his promotion of civil rights for blacks in the South. He especially hated Robert Kennedy, describing him as one of the three men he hated most in the world. [32–34] *

When Kennedy became President in 1961, he appointed his brother Robert to be Attorney General, making him Hoover's direct boss. Robert Kennedy installed an intercom and buzzer between their offices, irking Hoover immensely. [35] Hoover hated Robert Kennedy's meddling in the affairs of the FBI, particularly his contacting FBI agents and Bureau chiefs without first having secured Hoover's permission. Robert Kennedy circumvented Hoover for organized crime investigations, employing staff outside of the Director's control. [36]

It does not take much speculation to conclude that Hoover probably detested President Kennedy's charm and vigor with women. They swooned for JFK, and at the end of the day the photogenic Kennedys would both go home to their loving wives and children. The curmudgeonly Hoover would not.

President Kennedy undoubtedly resented Hoover's blackmail and use

---

known history of heart problems.

* The three men Hoover hated most in the world were Robert Kennedy, Martin Luther King, Jr., and Quinn Tamm, Director of the International Association of Chiefs of Police.

of federal police resources to constantly spy on his dalliances while in the White House. Eventually it came to be understood that after the 1964 election Hoover would be fired – that Hoover's dream of being FBI Director-for-Life would be shattered if JFK remained President.

Hoover's days as tyrannical dictator of the "Seat of Government", Hoover's name for the Bureau, would come to an end.

Instead, Kennedy was killed, and in January 1964, two months after the assassination, President Johnson held a lavish ceremony in the White House Rose Garden in which he praised Hoover as "a hero to millions of decent citizens, and an anathema to evil men", and announced that he had just signed an Executive Order exempting Hoover from compulsory retirement.

With Kennedy's death Hoover's dream of being the FBI's Director-for-Life had come to fruition.

CHAPTER 11

LYNDON JOHNSON, CORRUPT, MURDEROUS POLITICIAN

As midnight November 21st, 1963 quietly turned into the 22nd, Lyndon Johnson was a man in deep trouble.

His corrupt and murderous past was catching up to him, and there was a steady drumbeat of whispers that he would be dumped from the Presidential ticket and wind up in jail. But by midnight the next day, all of that was gone, all of those troubles had disappeared into the mist.

President Kennedy's murder had solved everything for Lyndon Johnson.

Johnson's troubles centered on two separate scandals that were coming to a boil, but his entire past in politics had been a history of lies, bribery, and murder. Johnson became infamous in 1948 by stuffing the ballot box in Alice, Texas, to produce a recount that favored him 200 to 1, thus handing him a seat in the U.S. Senate. [1]

In 1951 Johnson's preferred triggerman, Malcolm Wallace, was arrested, tried and convicted of killing a professional golfer named John Kinser. Kinser was having affairs with Wallace's wife and Johnson's sister, Josepha. Josepha was a promiscuous drug user who was thought to be revealing too much about Johnson's unsavory activities. After Wallace was convicted of first degree murder, Johnson prevailed upon the court to issue a suspended sentence of five years. [2] Johnson was later accused of having his sister Josepha killed.

One of Johnson's partners in corrupt dealings, Billy Sol Estes, eventually implicated him in numerous murders, including the murder of Henry Marshall by Malcolm Wallace. Marshall was an Agriculture Department official who had run afoul of the Johnson machine in 1961 by questioning cotton allotments that were used by Estes to finance Johnson. The trail uncovered by Marshall's investigation was leading inexorably to Johnson.

Then Vice President Johnson's apparent solution was to have Marshall murdered.

In June 1961 Marshall's body was found in a remote corner of his farm, with a hose leading from the tailpipe of his truck to the passenger compartment. He had been bludgeoned and shot five times with a bolt action rifle.

His death was declared a suicide. [3]

In grand jury proceedings in 1984 Billy Sol Estes openly accused Johnson of masterminding nine murders: [4]

1. John Kinser

2. Henry Marshall

3. George Krutilek

4. Ike Rogers and his secretary

5. Harold Orr

6. Coleman Wade

7. Josepha Johnson

8. President John Kennedy*

Johnson's second scandal originated with his protégé, Bobby Baker, who held an official position as Senate Secretary to the Majority Leader at a time when Lyndon Johnson was the Majority Leader of the Senate. Baker became bagman for Johnson's corrupt schemes, and in 1963 formal testimony in federal court tied Baker and his associates to payoffs from defense contractors that were destined for Johnson. [6]

Baker was also a founder of the Quorum Club, an elite social club near the Capitol that attracted powerful politicians and eventually became

* An unidentified fingerprint in the National Archives that was found on a cardboard box in the sixth floor sniper's nest was eventually traced to Malcolm Wallace, leading many to speculate that Wallace was the sixth floor shooter, or had been present on the sixth floor during the assassination. [5]

enmeshed in a prostitution for political favors scandal. [7]

Baker found himself entangled in a third scandal involving the Serv-U Corporation, a company set up to provide service for vending machines located in federal buildings. [8]

With the arrival of the Baker and Estes scandals Johnson found himself being slowly drawn into a swamp of political scandal from which there was little hope of escape, barring the death of the President and an end to the investigations. Johnson would complain vehemently that Robert Kennedy was out to get him through Kennedy's efforts to prosecute Baker and his associates, but after the President's death Johnson was in a position to shut down the investigations, which is exactly what happened. [9, 10]

In the course of events, knowledgeable insiders such as E. Howard Hunt and Billy Sol Estes have named Johnson as Kennedy's killer. They were eventually joined by Johnson's mistress, Madeleine Brown, who also bore Johnson's child. She stated that at Clint Murchison's party the night before the assassination Johnson told her that Kennedy would be killed. Johnson's threat came just after he emerged from a meeting that included Clint Murchison, J. Edgar Hoover, and Richard Nixon:

"Those Kennedys will never embarrass me again.

That's no threat, that's a promise."

It was repeated in a telephone call the next morning. [11, 12]

In 1979 the manager for Ronald Reagan's New York campaign for President, Roger Stone, set up a meeting with lawyer Roy Cohn to discuss support for Reagan. At the meeting Cohn and Mafia crime boss Anthony "Fat Tony" Salerno indicated that Carlos Marcello and Lyndon Johnson had killed Kennedy. [13] Johnson himself had substantial connections to organized crime figures, including Marcello; Robert Kennedy had assembled a considerable investigative file concerning the details of these relationships. [14]

Johnson's suspect behavior after the assassination also links him to the killing. Immediately after the assassination Johnson ordered the Presidential limousine to be sent back to Detroit for a complete refurbishing, removing all traces of critical forensic evidence that could explain how the President was killed. Johnson aide Cliff Carter ordered John Connally's clothing to be sent to the cleaners, again removing all traces of critical forensic evidence. [15]

Carter also phoned Dallas District Attorney Henry Wade and ordered him not allege a conspiracy in the prosecution of Oswald. Oswald was to be charged with simple murder, and was not to be associated with any kind of a conspiracy. [16, 17]

Johnson eventually issued Executive Order 11652, ensuring that the bulk of assassination evidence and documentation would be locked away in the National Archives, where it would remain far from public scrutiny until 2039. [18]

LYNDON JOHNSON,
THE ORIGINAL ANTHONY WEINER*

In the 1960s most Americans were unfamiliar with Lyndon Johnson's corrupt past and his potential involvement in the assassination. To many President Johnson was a courtly, grandfatherly figure, a man given to telling others how much he loved and appreciated them.

But history has shown that there was a darker, stranger side to Johnson, a side that caused him to engage in compulsive sexual exhibitionism.

Johnson frequently let it be known that he was quite proud of his penis, nicknaming it "Jumbo".[19] As a result, the term "Johnson" entered the American lexicon as a slang term for penis, slang that persists to this day.

Johnson was famous for his naked Cabinet meetings in the White House pool. He would break up Cabinet meetings by ordering his entire Cabinet, all male, to go to the White House pool, undress, and jump into the water. [20]

His all male shenanigans would continue in front of male reporters. Johnson would order them to his room, undress completely in front of them, and then get dressed again. Johnson's male striptease shows were well known to White House reporters. [21]

When reporters persistently questioned Johnson as to why the U.S. was in Vietnam, Johnson once unzipped his pants, took out his penis, and exclaimed, "This is why!".[22] Johnson was also well known for his indiscrete public urination, and for the display of his penis to other men in the men's

---

* Anthony Weiner is a New York City and federal politician famous for his compulsive sexual exhibitionism.

room. [23]

While in the Senate Johnson became infamous for his personal lobbying techniques, which collectively came to be known as the "Johnson treatment". The "Johnson treatment" consisted primarily of administrative threats, as well as Johnson physically leaning into other legislators to get his way. At 6' 4" Lyndon Johnson was a physically imposing man and was unafraid to use his size to intimidate others. Johnson's Vice President Hubert Humphrey once described a meeting with Johnson where he "came out of that session covered with blood, sweat, tears, spit - and sperm." [24]

It might be said that Lyndon Johnson was a man with a reputation.

CHAPTER 12

HOMOSEXUALITY AND
THE KENNEDY ASSASSINATION

WALTER JENKINS

Lyndon Johnson's habit of waving his penis around and exposing himself to other men in the men's room probably caught the attention of his closest aide, Walter Jenkins. Jenkins was Johnson's Chief of Staff and the second most powerful man in the White House. Jenkins had been Johnson's trusted aide for 25 years, and Johnson referred to him as "my vice president in charge of everything". [1, 2] Two days after the assassination an article in the Washington Post stated that "Figuratively speaking, Jenkins is always at Johnson's elbow." [3]

Following the assassination, Jenkins became Johnson's liaison to J. Edgar Hoover, maintaining the many sexual blackmail files that Hoover sent over to the White House. Like Hoover, Johnson had no reservations about contacting key politicians and letting it be known that the FBI had files and documentation concerning their sexual indiscretions. Everything would remain quiet as long as their cooperation could be ensured. [4]

Johnson, Hoover, and Jenkins thus became the three most powerful men in America, capable of controlling America's most powerful politicians and political destiny through the use of Hoover's sexual blackmail.

All of this came crashing to an end on October 7, 1964, when Walter Jenkins was arrested in the basement of the YMCA a few blocks from the White House. Jenkins had been observed by two plainclothes policemen performing oral sex on a retired Army sergeant in a pay toilet stall. [5]

Jenkins' arrest only a few weeks before the 1964 Presidential election came at a very inopportune time for Lyndon Johnson. Johnson and his team

did their best to suppress the information from leaking out to the press. After a week the story became public knowledge and scandal ensued. [6] *
Johnson's media team claimed that Jenkins had cracked under the stress of the campaign, but that explanation was undermined by the fact that Jenkins had been arrested for exactly the same offense in exactly the same location five years previously. [10]

Jenkins had also been accused by a park policeman of attempted solicitation in LaFayette Park prior to his second arrest at the YMCA. Johnson asked the FBI to bring pressure on the policeman concerning the accusation. [11]

It's hard to imagine that Johnson did not know about Jenkins' previous legal problems or his homosexual desires, and in fact a more likely scenario is that Johnson had his own "man-love" desires, not necessarily in the sense of frequenting homosexual establishments or similar environments, but more likely that of demanding sexual tribute from his subordinates in return for his good favor. In his mind Lyndon Johnson was the alpha male and he obviously wanted everyone else to know, understand, and acknowledge that.

One can only imagine what might have occurred during Oval Office meetings involving Lyndon "Jumbo" Johnson, Edgar "Red Dress" Hoover, and Walter "YMCA" Jenkins. Surely this could be one of America's most

---

* The discovery of Walter Jenkins as a closet homosexual soon precipitated a witch hunt for homosexuals in the Johnson administration. Word among the Republicans was that Johnson had a homosexual in his cabinet. Suspicion soon fell on Johnson's newly hired Special Assistant, Jack Valenti, who was present at Johnson's side when Johnson was sworn in as President in Dallas. Valenti had to defend himself against charges that he had overnight stays with a homosexual photographer. J. Edgar Hoover, however, vouched for Valenti, and Valenti was allowed to continue on in his position. Many nonetheless thought that Valenti was gay. Valenti was president of the of the Motion Picture Association of America from 1966 through 2004, and presided over the liberalization of Hollywood's attitude toward homosexuality.[7,8] The FBI in fact identified two members of Johnson's cabinet who were thought to have been homosexual.[9] There was also substantial discussion in the press about the propriety of Hoover's having sent Jenkins a bouquet of flowers in the hospital following his arrest.

tightly held secrets.

What are the odds that the three most powerful men in America were homosexuals due solely to chance? If the frequently cited Kinsey figure of 10% for male homosexuality is used, the odds are 1 in 1,000. If the current Center for Disease Control estimate of 2% is used, the odds become even longer at 1 in 125,000. [12]

Based on these statistics, the conclusion may be drawn that after the Kennedy assassination the three most powerful men in America were sexually connected to each other, and that the presence of three such sexually extreme individuals at the pinnacle of power in America was no accident. And if they were connected this way after the assassination, they were most likely connected this way before the assassination.

CLAY SHAW AND DAVID FERRIE

In the film *JFK* both Clay Shaw and David Ferrie are accurately portrayed as homosexuals. Clay Shaw was well known within the New Orleans homosexual community, and it was his contacts there that enabled Jim Garrison to track him down from the alias "Clay Betrand" provided by lawyer Dean Andrews. Ferrie had been arrested for homosexual pedophilia and dismissed from his job as a pilot for Eastern Airlines. One scene in the film shows Shaw and Ferrie at a homosexual party, a depiction based on photographs taken at an actual gay party in New Orleans.

The portrayal of Shaw and Ferrie as homosexuals brought predictable howls of outrage from the homosexual left. That Shaw and Ferrie were in fact homosexual is beyond dispute, but according to the argument, scenes depicting their homosexuality were gratuitously added to the film solely to demonize homosexuals as sinister murderers – their homosexuality had nothing to do with JFK's murder and should not have been included in the film. [13]

Further analysis, however, shows that the presence of homosexuals at the visible edges of the assassination is more substantial than just Shaw and Ferrie, and extends to include Jack Ruby and Lee Harvey Oswald. In fact, the operational arm of the assassination that runs from Permindex and Clay Shaw through Oswald consists of four homosexuals: Shaw, Ferrie, Ruby,

189

and Oswald. Only the CIA-associated stage managers of that arm, such as Guy Banister, appear to have been straight.

To this day the homosexual left still insists that Clay Shaw was the victim of anti-homosexual prejudice by Jim Garrison. The argument advanced is that Garrison learned from Dean Andrews' Warren Commission testimony that Andrews had been contacted by an individual named Clay Bertrand immediately after the assassination to represent Lee Harvey Oswald, and that "Bertrand" was a homosexual who referred homosexual clients to Andrews.

Garrison, it is alleged, focused on and prosecuted a completely innocent Clay Shaw solely because Shaw was a homosexual with the same first name as "Clay Bertrand".

This analysis, however, does not withstand reasonable scrutiny. Clay Shaw was connected to the CIA and performed contract work for the CIA. The CIA monitored Shaw's trial in New Orleans and provided assistance on his behalf. Clay Shaw was a director of Permindex, an international corporation connected to assassinations. [14]

Garrison knew none of this when he investigated and prosecuted Shaw for conspiracy to assassinate the President, becoming aware of these facts only after the trial.

To suggest that Garrison prosecuted Shaw solely because he was homosexual is to imply that Shaw's connections to the CIA and Permindex were all just an enormous coincidence, when in essence these connections serve to validate Garrison's investigation after the fact.

JACK RUBY

The Warren Commission went to great lengths to tell America that Jack Ruby was not homosexual:

"There have been statements that Ruby was a homosexual. The available evidence does not support the allegation. There is no evidence of homosexuality on his part; Ruby did not frequent known gathering places for homosexuals, many of the reports were inherently suspect or based upon questionable or inaccurate premises, and Ruby and most of his associates and employees denied the charge. All the allegations were based on hearsay or derive from Ruby's lisp or a 'feeling' that Ruby was a 'sissy,' seemed 'weird,' acted effeminately, and sometimes spoke in a high pitched voice when angry…" [15]

A different story, however, hides in plain sight in the back pages of the reports of the Warren Commission and House Select Committee on Assassinations. The Commission was correct in stating that the impression many had that Ruby was homosexual was not based on first-hand knowledge. At the time of the assassination Ruby was living with a man named George Senator. Ruby's employee Larry Crafard felt that Senator was homosexual. Senator liked to introduce Ruby as his "boyfriend", but coyly denied to the Warren Commission that he was gay, stating that "Georgie still loves women yet". [16]

The FBI interviewed one witness whose name was found on a Ruby notepad. She stated that the friend who introduced her to Ruby also provided cash register servicing to Ruby's club, and that that individual felt that "Jack liked boys". [17] Others described hearing rumors that Ruby was homosexual. [18]

The Secret Service eventually received word that a Texas stripper named Helen K. Smith, who performed under the name "Dixie Lynn", had information indicating that Jack Ruby and Lee Harvey Oswald attended the same homosexual parties in Dallas. Smith was interviewed by Dallas Police Officer Lieutenant Jack Revill. At the interview Smith appeared to be upset because she recognized Revill as part of a previous narcotics investigation that convicted a stripper friend of hers. Smith denied having attended any party at which Jack Ruby or Lee Harvey Oswald was present.

Subsequent investigation determined that the source of the information was a bartender at the Midnight Lounge in Houston, Travis Binkendorfer, who repeated Smith's story to investigators, and mentioned that according to Smith a Dallas attorney named Barbara Welz had also attended the party. Binkendorfer had served as a police informant in the past. [19]

According to some, both Jack Ruby and Lee Harvey Oswald made appearances at gay hangouts (Figure 12-1).

Carlos Marcello, the Mafia godfather of Louisiana and Texas, thought that Ruby was gay. Marcello stated to an FBI informant that "Ruby was a homo son of a bitch but good to have around to report…what was happening

```
FD-302 (Rev. 3-3-59)          FEDERAL BUREAU OF INVESTIGATION
      1

                                                Date  11/27/63

           ROBERT KERMIT PATTERSON, commonly known as BOB
      PATTERSON, appeared at the Dallas Field Division on November
      2?, 1963.  PATTERSON advised that he resides in Room 511
      at the YMCA located at 605 North Ervay Street, Dallas,
      Texas.  PATTERSON advised that at the present time he is
      a student at the Metropolitan Technical Institute, 402 North
      Good-Latimer, Dallas, Texas.

           According to PATTERSON, he was born on January 24, 1930,
      at Lincoln, Nebraska, and had the rating of RD-3 while in
      the U. S. Navy.  His U. S. Navy Serial Number is 4278665.

           PATTERSON informed that he is a homosexual and as
      such has access to the so-called "gay" bars and lounges in
      the City of Dallas, Texas.  He said that although he has only
      been in Dallas for approximately two years he is acquainted
      with many of the "gay" people in Dallas.

           PATTERSON stated that on the evening of November
      26, 1963, he was at one of the "gay" spots in town,
      specifically The Villa-Fontana, 1315 Skiles.  PATTERSON said
      that he was broke and prevailed upon JERRY, the bartender
      at the Villa-Fontana, to set up some beer for him.  While
      at the bar drinking, JERRY, the bartender, introduced him to
      another chap named JERRY, who was also sitting at the bar.
      JERRY, the bartender, who is a member of the "gay" set
      in Dallas, vouched for PATTERSON's standing with the "gay"
      set to the other JERRY, and the conversation thereupon flowed
      freely.  During the conversation, the unknown JERRY, the customer,
      whom PATTERSON described as about 33 years old, heavy set,
      approximately 5 feet 7 inches, dark hair and round face,
      made the statement that he is the former lover of JACK
      RUBY.  PATTERSON also heard one or the other of the JERRYs
      mention that GEORGE SENATOR, roommate of JACK RUBY's at
      the time of RUBY's arrest, was also a "gay" person.

           PATTERSON likewise stated that he heard it mentioned
      at the Villa-Fontana on November 26, 1963, that LEE HARVEY
      OSWALD had been seen at the Holiday Bar and also in Gene's
      Music Bar, both of which PATTERSON described as hangouts
      for the "gay" crowd.

─────────────────────────────────────────────────────────────────

on  11/27/63  at    Dallas, Texas            File #    DL 44-1639
                                                        89-43
by Special Agent   JOHN J. FLANAGAN/csh        Date dictated  11/27/63

This document contains neither recommendations nor conclusions of the FBI. It is the property of the FBI and is loaned to
your agency; it and its contents are not to be distributed outside your agency.
```

Figure 12-1. Page 1 of Warren Commission Exhibit 3013. [20]

in town." [21, 22]

One of Ruby's last phone calls was to entertainer Breck Wall. Ruby called Wall in Galveston around midnight on November 23, 1963, a few hours before he murdered Oswald in the basement of police headquarters. [23] It may be recalled that David Ferrie went to Galveston after the assassination, stopping along the way at an ice skating rink in Houston to make phone calls.

In his Warren Commission testimony Wall described himself as a close friend of Ruby: "I was Jack's best friend. I was the only one allowed in jail to see him." [24]

Wall eventually rose to fame as the producer of flamboyant male transvestite shows in Las Vegas. Wall felt that he had been hounded by New Orleans District Attorney Jim Garrison because of his homosexuality, but was relieved after the FBI absolved him of culpability in the assassination.*

No less an authority on homosexuality than J. Edgar Hoover himself pronounced Ruby to be homosexual:

---

* Wall was president of the American Guild of Variety Artists union. In his Warren Commission testimony Wall stated that he went to Galveston along with his friend and business partner, Joe Patterson, to visit his adoptive parents, Mr. and Mrs. Tom McKenna, and that it was there that he received a phone call from Jack Ruby. [25] He testified that Ruby called to discuss Ruby's union problems, but if assertions that Ruby and Oswald were homosexual lovers are true, a more likely scenario would have been to discuss the potential impact of Oswald's arrest on their circle of friends. With regard to Garrison's investigation, Wall could very well have been the innocent victim of circumstances, namely that i) he was Jack Ruby's self-proclaimed best friend, ii) he drove to Galveston at exactly the same time David Ferrie did, and iii) he received a telephone call from Ruby a few hours before Ruby murdered Oswald. Galveston appears in Rose Cheramie's account as a transfer point for a large quantity of heroin around the time Kennedy was assassinated, which could explain the reason for Ferrie's trip (Appendix III).

FACSIMILE

November 24, 1963

Mr. J. Edgar Hoover said as follows:

...They brought him (Oswald) out of the City Jail and were taking him to the County Jail when a man stepped out and shot him in the stomach. This man was arrested at once. He goes under the name of Jack Leon Ruby but his real name is Rubenstein. He runs two night clubs in Dallas and has the reputation of being a homosexual...[26]

LEE HARVEY OSWALD

On the face of it, it might seem unlikely that Lee Harvey Oswald was homosexual. He had a wife and two children, and testimony exists indicating that Oswald had expressed an interest in Japanese women while stationed in Japan. [27]

However, the pages of the Warren Commission Report tell a different story. When New Orleans attorney Dean Andrews appeared before the Warren Commission, he talked about how Oswald was sent to him by "Clay Bertrand", an alias used by Clay Shaw:

Mr. Liebeler: I am advised by the FBI that you told them that Lee Harvey Oswald came into your office some time during the summer of 1963. Would you tell us in your own words just what happened as far as that is concerned?

Mr. Andrews: I don't recall the dates, but briefly, it is this: Oswald came in the office accompanied by some gay kids. They were Mexicanos. He wanted to find out what could be done in connection with a discharge...

Mr. Liebeler: The first time he came in he was with these Mexicans,

194

and there were also some gay kids. By that, of course, you mean people that appeared to you to be homosexuals?

Mr. Andrews: Well, they swish. What they are, I don't know. We call them gay kids…

Mr. Liebeler: You say that some of the gay kids that you saw at the time the police arrested this large group of them for wearing clothes of the opposite sex were the ones that had been with Oswald?

Mr. Andrews: Yes…

Mr. Liebeler: I suppose the New Orleans Police Department files would reflect the dates these people were picked up?

Mr. Andrews: I checked the first district's blotter and the people are there, but I just can't get their names. You see, they wear names just like you and I wear clothes. Today their name is Candy; tomorrow it is Butsie; next day it is Mary. You never know what they are. Names are a very improbable method of identification…Only time I really paid attention to this boy (Oswald), he was in the front of the Maison Blanche Building giving out these kooky Castro things.

Mr. Liebeler: When was this approximately?

Mr. Andrews: I don't remember. I was coming from the NBC building, and I walked past him. You know how you see somebody, recognize him. So I turned around, came back, and asked him what he was doing giving that junk out. He said it was a job. I reminded him of the $25 he owed the office. He said he would come over there, but he never did.

Mr. Liebeler: Did he tell you that he was getting paid to hand out this literature?

Mr. Andrews: Yes…

Mr. Liebeler: Now what can you tell us about this Clay Bertrand? You met him prior to that time?

Mr. Andrews: I had seen Clay Bertrand once some time ago, probably a couple of years. He's the one who calls in behalf of gay kids normally, either to obtain bond or parole for them. I would assume that he was the one that originally sent Oswald and the gay kids, these Mexicanos, to the office because I had never seen those people before at all. They were just walk-ins.

Mr. Liebeler: You say that you think you saw Clay Bertrand some time about 2 years prior to the time you received this telephone call that you have just told us about?

Mr. Andrews: Yes; he is mostly a voice on the phone.

Mr. Liebeler: What day did you receive the telephone call from Clay Bertrand asking you to defend Oswald?

Mr. Andrews: I don't remember. It was a Friday or Saturday.

Mr. Liebeler: Immediately following the assassination?

Mr. Andrews: I don't know about that. I didn't know. Yes; I did. I guess I did because I was – they told me that I was squirrelly in the hospital.

Mr. Liebeler: You had pneumonia; is that right?

Mr. Andrews: Yes.

Mr. Liebeler: And as I understand it, you were under heavy sedation at the time in connection with your treatment for pneumonia?

Mr. Andrews: Yes, this is what happened: After I got the call, I called my secretary at her home and asked her if she had remembered Lee Harvey Oswald's file. Of course, she didn't remember, and I had to

196

tell her about all the kooky kids. She thought we had a file in the office. I would assume that he would have called subsequent to this boy's arrest. I am pretty sure it was before the assassination. I don't know.

Mr. Liebeler: You don't mean before the assassination – don't you mean before Oswald had been shot? After the assassination and before Oswald had been shot?

Mr. Andrews: After Oswald's arrest and prior to his -

Mr. Liebeler: His death?

Mr. Andrews: His death...

Mr. Liebeler: Has this fellow Bertrand sent you business in the past?

Mr. Andrews: Prior to – I guess the last time would be February of 1963.

Mr. Liebeler: And mostly he refers, I think you said, these gay kids, is that right?

Mr. Andrews: Right...

Mr. Liebeler: Did Oswald appear to you to be gay?

Mr. Andrews: You can't tell. I couldn't say. He swang with the kids. He didn't swish, but birds of a feather flock together. I don't know any squares that run with them...but I just assumed that he knew these people and was running with them. They had no reason to come. The three gay kids he was with, they were ostentatious. They were what we call swishers...I have no way of telling whether he is gay or not, other than he came in with what they call here queens. That's about it. [28]

Andrews made similar remarks testifying before the Grand Jury convened by Jim Garrison in New Orleans:

Q: … All right – would you tell us …

A: A voice that I identify as Clay Bertrand called me at the hospital and asked me if I would represent Lee Oswald in Dallas – nobody ever asked me about a fee or anything else – he said I would get real famous and he would get in touch with Lee Oswald so that I could represent him…

Q: I am sure you have these things you mention plaguing your memory, but my question is that you recognized Clay Bertrand's voice over the telephone, …

A: I talked to him about 10 or 12 times.

Q: All right. Will you tell the gentlemen the nature of your conversations with him?

A: He guaranteed payment for whatever services I was performing for whatever people called.

Q: That is rather broad – is it a particular category of people, or …

A: They were gay people.

Q: You mean homosexuals? That you represented?

A: Man, they bat off both sides of the plate – I don't know what they do – I don't keep score – they just walk in the office. [29]

Others in New Orleans felt that Oswald was homosexual. Anti-Castro Cuban refugee leader Santos Miguel Gonzalez stated that Oswald was well known among the New Orleans Cuban exile community as both an *agent provocateur* and a homosexual. [30]

Homosexual pedophile David Ferrie was Oswald's commanding officer in the Civil Air Patrol when Oswald was an impressionable boy of sixteen. Ferrie was dismissed from the Air Patrol when it was discovered that he was organizing nude drinking parties with some of the teenaged boys. The Warren Commission and its supporters long maintained that there was no connection between Ferrie and Oswald, until photographs surfaced showing the two together at Civil Air Patrol gatherings. [31]

Some of Oswald's comrades in the Marines believed him to be homosexual. Daniel Powers, a fellow marine at Keesler Air Force Base, stated that he thought Oswald to be homosexual because Oswald had a lot of "feminine characteristics". Marine David Christie also felt that Oswald was gay. Oswald reportedly visited a transvestite bar in Japan, and a gay bar called the Flamingo in Tijuana, Mexico, while serving in the Marines in California. [32]

Recently former Governor Jesse Ventura published further details about Oswald's homosexuality. Military Intelligence analyst Jim Southwood described receiving a request in September 1962 from the 112th Military Intelligence Group for information concerning Oswald and George de Mohrenschildt. He replied that "Oswald was a peculiar guy, that he had strange sexual practices…", and that Army and Naval intelligence in Japan determined that "he'd been known to frequent homosexual bars. One of the reports was that he was suspected of being involved in a homosexual relationship with a Soviet colonel." Southwood went on to relate how the Deputy Director of the CIA, General Marshall Carter, had an intense interest in Oswald. [33]

In some assassination scenarios Oswald's marital difficulties played a central role in his decision to kill the President. Oswald's wife would complain that she was being sexually neglected by Oswald, and she accused him of not being a man.[34] The theory advanced by many Warren Commission supporters is that Oswald killed the President to compensate for his lack of manhood and shortcomings as a husband.

The appearance of numerous homosexuals in the operational arm of the assassination did not escape the attention of New Orleans District Attorney Jim Garrison. Garrison determined that Shaw, Ferrie, Ruby, and Oswald were all homosexuals. In the initial phase of his investigation Garrison thought that the assassination had been a "homosexual thrill killing". [35]

It is of interest to note that the anonymous Torbitt document declared that the upper and lower echelons of the assassination consisted of "sexual deviates". The term "sexual deviate" as used in the 1960s and 70s typically referred to homosexuals.

DID OSWALD AND RUBY KNOW EACH OTHER?

In addition to assuring America that Jack Ruby was not gay, the Warren Commission also stated that Ruby and Lee Harvey Oswald did not know each other:

"The Commission made intensive inquiry into the backgrounds and relationships of Oswald and Ruby to determine whether they knew each other or were involved in a plot of any kind with each other or others. It was unable to find any credible evidence to support the rumors linking Oswald and Ruby directly or through others. The Commission concluded that they were not involved in a conspiratorial relationship with each other or with any third parties." [36]

Speculation. – Ruby and Oswald were seen together at the Carousel Club.

Commission Finding. – All assertions that Oswald was seen in the company of Ruby or of anyone else at the Carousel Club have been investigated. None of them merits any credence. [37]

Speculation. – Oswald was on his way to Jack Ruby's apartment when he was stopped by Patrolman Tippit.

Commission Finding. – There is no evidence that Oswald and Ruby knew each other or had any relationship through a third party or parties. There is no evidence that Oswald knew where Ruby lived. Accordingly, there is neither evidence nor reason to believe that Oswald was on his way to Ruby's apartment when he was stopped by Tippit. [38]

The facts, however, present a different picture. Oswald's mother, Marguerite Oswald, testified before the Warren Commission that after her son was apprehended the FBI showed her a picture of Jack Ruby, and asked if she knew him, thus indicating that the FBI had already connected Oswald and Ruby well before Ruby's attack in the police headquarters basement. [39]

A day after the assassination a witness reported a truck parked near the grassy knoll an hour before Kennedy's arrival. The witness claimed afterward that the police showed her a photo of Ruby, and asked if he was the driver. [40]

After Ruby shot Oswald there was rampant press speculation that the two knew each other (Figure 12-2). A National Enquirer article stated that "Dallas cops suspected Oswald of being the gunman and Ruby the paymaster in a plot to murder former Major General Edwin A. Walker seven months before the President was assassinated" and that "the Justice Department deliberately kept Oswald and Ruby out of jail before the assassination." It went on to assert that "the U.S. Central Intelligence Agency was using Ruby to recruit commandos for raids against Castro's Cuba" and that "a

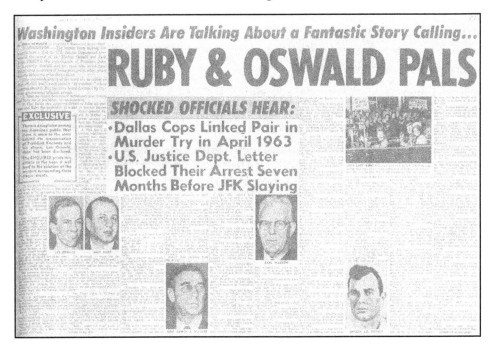

Figure 12-2. Warren Commission Exhibit 837 concerning press speculation about the relationship between Jack Ruby and Lee Harvey Oswald.

letter signed by a high official of the Justice Dept. was sent in April 1963 from the Justice Dept. to Dallas Chief of Police Jesse E. Curry requesting the Dallas police not to arrest Oswald and Ruby in connection with the attempted slaying of General Walker."

It is well established that Ruby attended a press conference that took place around midnight the evening of the assassination. Dallas District Attorney Henry Wade was asked if Oswald was a member of any Communist front organizations. Wade mentioned the "Free Cuba Movement", which Ruby immediately corrected to "Fair Play for Cuba". Only ten hours after Oswald's capture Ruby had displayed a detailed knowledge of Oswald's pre-assassination activities.

After Ruby shot Oswald, the Master of Ceremonies at Ruby's Carousel Club was interviewed by Dan Rather on national television. He stated that he had seen Oswald in the club the week before.[41] Beverly Oliver, who worked in the adjacent Colony Club, said that Ruby introduced Oswald to her as "my friend Lee". Oliver felt that "Lee Harvey Oswald and Jack Ruby were linked together" in some manner.[42] That sentiment was echoed in a newspaper interview with Ruby stripper Jada Conforto. Lyndon Johnson's mistress, Madeleine Brown, worked for a period of time at the Carousel Club. She maintained that she had seen Oswald at the club, and that there was a direct link between Oswald and Ruby.[43, 44] Carousel Club performers Bill Demar, Wally Weston, and Karen Carlin all stated that they had seen Oswald at the club. [45]

Perhaps one of the most interesting stories about Ruby is that of Rose Cheramie (also spelled Cherami). Cheramie was a prostitute and heroin addict who was found lying injured in the road near Eunice, Louisiana, on November 20, 1963. She was taken to the Louisiana State Hospital for treatment of her injuries and narcotics withdrawal. At the hospital she told the attending physician that President Kennedy would be killed on his upcoming trip to Dallas. Her assertions were ignored as the rantings of a heroin addict suffering from withdrawal. After the assassination the State Police were called and she was questioned in detail about her allegations.

Cheramie said that she worked as a stripper in Ruby's night club. She referred to Ruby as "Pinky". She stated that she had seen Oswald at the club, that Oswald and Ruby knew each other well, and that in fact Oswald and Ruby were homosexual lovers. She further stated that "word in the underworld" was that Kennedy would be assassinated. She was found dead two years later after being run over on a Texas highway. The House Select Committee investigation of Rose Cheramie's claims is contained in Appendix III.*

Another curious facet of the assassination is the strange path that Oswald took after he left the Texas School Book Depository. The Warren Commission maintained that after Kennedy was killed, Oswald took a bus, and then a cab. The Dallas Morning News published an article on November 28, 1963 in which cab driver Bill Whaley stated that Oswald asked him to go to 500 North Beckley (the Warren Commission later revised this to 700 North Beckley, two blocks closer to Oswald's residence).[46] This destination took Oswald about 800 yards past his rooming house, and approximately halfway to Jack Ruby's apartment (Figure 12-3). After exiting the cab, Oswald reversed direction, returned home, and retrieved his revolver. He then continued on his original path south on Beckley. As shown in Figure 12-3 Oswald was heading towards Jack Ruby's apartment at the time he allegedly encountered Officer Tippit and killed him. [47]

* Rose Cherami's account is examined in detail in *A Rose By Many Other Names: Rose Cherami and the JFK Assassination* by Todd Elliott. Elliott worked as an investigative journalist for the *Eunice News*, a newspaper situated in the town where Cherami was first picked up. The title of the book derives from the fact that Cherami was known to have over 35 aliases.

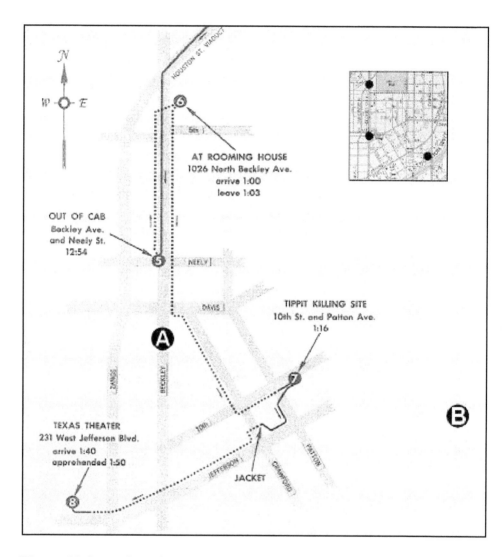

Figure 12-3. Portion of Warren Commission Exhibit 1119-A, "Whereabouts of Lee Harvey Oswald between 12:33 P.M. and 1:50 P.M. November 22, 1963", modified to show the original account of where Oswald exited Bill Whaley's cab at the 500 block of North Beckley (A) and the location of Jack Ruby's apartment (B). Inset: top circle, location of Oswald's rooming house; middle circle, Oswald's point of exiting the taxi; bottom circle, location of Jack Ruby's apartment.

CHAPTER 13

DID LEE HARVEY OSWALD SHOOT PRESIDENT KENNEDY?

νο

One of the central questions of the Kennedy assassination is whether Lee Harvey Oswald shot the President, or was he simply an innocent scapegoat destined for blame and execution by the real killers. Jim Garrison, for example, believed that Oswald was completely innocent of any involvement in the assassination, and was simply given assignments by his intelligence handlers, such as pro-Castro leafleting and radio speeches, to burnish his credentials as an ardent Communist for the day when he would be blamed for killing President Kennedy.*

The question of Oswald's guilt is quite complex due to a number of factors. The presence of high ranking CIA operative E. Howard Hunt in Dealey Plaza signals the possibility of CIA involvement and expertise in the President's murder. Prior to his deathbed confession Hunt denied being in Dealey Plaza during the assassination, and in fact claimed to have been at home in Washington. In 1978 Victor Marchetti wrote an article for the Liberty Lobby newspaper *Spotlight* alleging that the House Select Committee on Assassinations had obtained a 1966 CIA memorandum stating that CIA operatives E. Howard Hunt, Frank Sturgis, and Gerry Patrick Hemming had been involved in the assassination of the President.** The House Select Committee chose not to publish the memo.

Hunt sued Liberty Lobby for defamation and in 1981 was awarded

---

* According to attorney Dean Andrews' Warren Commission testimony, Oswald himself told Andrews that he was being paid to hand out pro-Castro leaflets, calling it a "job" (Andrews testimony, Chapter 12).
** Hemming was Oswald's Marine sergeant when Oswald was stationed at the top secret CIA U-2 base in Atsugi, Japan. [1]

$650,000 in damages. The verdict was overturned on appeal due to erroneous jury instructions concerning defamation law. Hunt sued again and Liberty Lobby retained lawyer Mark Lane for the second trial.

Lane used Hunt's defamation suit as an opportunity to put the CIA on trial. As a result of the discovery process and trial he was able to extract documentation and testimony that not only implied CIA involvement in Kennedy's death, but also demonstrated strenuous efforts by the CIA to mislead or otherwise exert pressure to influence the outcome of the Warren Commission and House Select Committee investigations. Lane and Liberty Lobby prevailed in the second trial, which became the basis for Lane's 1991 book, *Plausible Denial: Was the CIA Involved in the Assassination of JFK?*

The presence of the CIA in Dealey Plaza moves analysis of the Kennedy assassination into an entirely different universe, not only due to the CIA's killing expertise and skill in setting up assassinations, but also their renown as masters of disinformation and media manipulation, use of doubles and disguise, as well as the corruption of political and judicial systems through physical intimidation, force, or other means.

There are additional factors that complicate analysis of Oswald's potential guilt, and if guilty, who might have assisted or motivated him to fire on the President. Oswald, Ferrie, and Ruby were all homosexuals and it has been alleged that all three knew each other. All three had connections to CIA sponsored efforts to overthrow Fidel Castro.

It is also known that all three had connections to organized crime. Ruby was a well known representative and payoff man for the Mafia in Dallas, and he served to channel Mob funding for CIA inspired operations to remove Castro from power. Ferrie worked for New Orleans crime boss Carlos Marcello. Oswald as well had family connections to organized crime, and in particular, Carlos Marcello's criminal empire. His mother dated individuals connected to Marcello. His uncle and surrogate father, Charles Murret, was a bookie for Marcello's illegal gambling operations.[2, 3] An FBI informant stated that Marcello himself met Oswald at Marcello's brother's restaurant, in the company of David Ferrie. [4]

These diverse connections amongst Oswald, Ferrie, and Ruby complicate efforts to understand exactly what forces could have placed Oswald with a rifle on the sixth floor of the Texas School Book Depository shooting at the President.

While the authorities assembled a strong case against Oswald based on physical evidence and witness testimony, much of it could have been fabricated in an attempt to frame Oswald. The strongest case against Oswald, therefore, is marshaled by his unusual behavior the day before the assassination, and immediately afterward.

After starting work at the Texas School Book Depository in October 1963 Oswald established a pattern of living at a rooming house in Dallas during the week, and returning on weekends to his wife and children who were staying at Ruth Paine's house in Irving, a suburb of Dallas. He was given a ride to Dallas on Monday mornings, and a ride back to Irving on Friday afternoons, by his co-worker Buell Wesley Frazier, who was a neighbor of the Paines.

The day before the assassination Oswald requested that Frazier give him a ride back to Irving, ostensibly to pick up some curtain rods for his room in Dallas. According to the Warren Commission Report, when Oswald went to work the next morning he left his wedding ring on top of his dresser and a wallet containing $170 in a dresser drawer.

That morning Oswald carried a bulky package to work. Frazier estimated the package to be about two feet in length. The longest piece of the Mannlicher-Carcano rifle that Oswald allegedly used to shoot the President was approximately 2' 10" inches in length, and if stored diagonally in the package it would have had an effective length of approximately two and a half feet.

After the assassination Oswald took a cab past his rooming house and halfway to Jack Ruby's apartment. He exited the cab, doubled back to his rooming house where he retrieved his revolver and headed out again in the direction of Ruby's apartment. He was walking towards Ruby's residence with a loaded gun when he allegedly encountered Officer Tippit. [5]

It's hard to imagine Oswald's behavior as that of an innocent man. Common sense dictates that if Oswald was interested in installing curtain rods at his rooming house, he would have waited until the next day, a Friday, when his normal routine would have taken him back to Ruth Paine's house in Irving. His presence in Jack Ruby's neighborhood after the assassination with a loaded gun only serves to further arouse suspicion that he was, in fact, in some way involved in the assassination of the President.

What could have motivated Oswald to fire on the President? Money, and a pretext that he was doing the right thing for America.

Social psychologists have shown that it is easier to motivate an individual to perform an odious act that violates their conscience if a pretext is supplied that allows the individual to assign blame to someone else, particularly if that someone else is presented as an authority figure. In the case of Oswald, the pretext would have come from his intelligence handlers in the form of assertions that Kennedy was the dupe of Communists and a security threat, and therefore had to be removed from office for the good of America.

Who could have offered Oswald money? Jack Ruby, Mafia and CIA payoff man, and alleged bedmate of Oswald, seems like the most likely candidate.

And after Oswald was caught, what was Ruby's only alternative to avoid being killed by the Mafia as a man who knew too much? Shooting Oswald dead and winding up in the protection of a Dallas jail cell.

CHAPTER 14

WHO KILLED THE PRESIDENT?

The Seven Big Lies of the Medical Evidence were created to disguise the fact that President Kennedy was struck by more than two bullets, and that it was therefore impossible that Oswald acted alone. These obvious and outrageous lies were invented and promoted by well placed federal insiders such as Arlen Specter, David Belin, and Gerald Ford, and establish the central conclusion of the Kennedy assassination:

President Kennedy was assassinated as the result of a conspiracy that emanated, wholly or in part, from within the federal government of the United States. There is no other reason why employees of the federal government would attempt to cover up such a massive crime.*

What additional information can be obtained from other observable facts to form a general picture of events on November 22, 1963?

First, the President's body was already on the autopsy table when the casket allegedly bearing it arrived with his widow at the front door of the Bethesda Naval Medical Center. This observation, confirmed by individuals present at the autopsy, bears witness to an immense federal subterfuge underlying the assassination. It shows evidence of a highly

---

* Specter, Belin, and Ford all went on to have successful careers within the federal establishment. Specter became a U.S. senator, Belin was appointed to run the Rockefeller Commission, and Ford was appointed to the Presidency of the United States. This is in stark contrast to Warren Commissioner Hale Boggs, who expressed doubt about the Commission's single bullet theory. Boggs disappeared without a trace in a mysterious plane crash over Alaska.

disciplined, well oiled assassination machine, extensive planning, and highly motivated federal security insiders who ruthlessly executed their assigned tasks as specified by the assassination planners. An infamous video of the assassination shows a Secret Service agent standing on the back bumper of the President's limousine being waved off by a superior as it was about to depart the airport. The agent would have blocked the path of a rifle shot from the Texas School Book Depository. The Secret Service instructed the Dallas Police to position the President's motorcycle escort behind the Presidential limousine, and not abreast, as was usually the case for Presidential motorcades. Immediately after the assassination the Secret Service cleaned the interior of the President's limousine - at that moment the most important crime scene in American history - so as to obscure all traces of blood spatter and other important forensic evidence. The Secret Service failed to record or create a transcript of Oswald's interrogations. The Secret Service was the recipient of the original autopsy photos and X-rays that were eventually transformed into the transparently fraudulent autopsy exhibits deposited in the National Archives.*

Second, both the FBI and the Warren Commission had first rate investigative resources at their disposal, yet erroneously concluded that Jack Ruby had no significant link to organized crime. The House Select Committee on Assassinations found that Jack Ruby had extensive and obvious connections to organized crime. Ruby was the top payoff man for the Mob in Dallas, eventually coming to corrupt the entire Dallas Police Department and judicial apparatus. He was also a major player in funding CIA-backed efforts to topple Castro. Why would the FBI and Warren Commission look the other way when it came to Ruby's Mob connections? Why did the Warren Commission devote an entire paragraph to telling America that Ruby was not homosexual, when all available evidence was to the contrary?

Third, Mafia figures had advance knowledge of the assassination. Jack Ruby, Carlos Marcello, and Santos Trafficante all exhibited knowledge in advance that President Kennedy was going to be killed. Santos Trafficante in particular stated before the assassination that "Kennedy's not going to

---

* It is well known that the head of the Secret Service at the time of the assassination, James Rowley, was a good friend of Lyndon Johnson, as well as J. Edgar Hoover, his former boss. [1]

make the election. He's going to be hit." Robert Blakey, General Counsel for the House Select Committee on Assassinations, contended that President Kennedy was killed as the result of a "Mob hit". A "Mob hit", however, could not explain why certain federal insiders would create and certify such a massive and obvious fraud concerning the medical evidence of the President's wounds. The differing positions of Blakey and Garrison on the assassination eventually degenerated into a literary shouting match, with Blakey supporters stating that Garrison purposefully ignored the participation of Carlos Marcello in the assassination, and Garrison supporters claiming that Blakey deliberately ignored the participation of individuals connected to the CIA.

Blakey's theory of a "Mob hit" centered largely around the activities of New Orleans godfather Carlos Marcello, whose criminal empire stretched well into Louisiana and Texas. Marcello was eventually incarcerated and at one point federal prison officials observed him talking about "getting" President Kennedy in Dallas. After publicly cursing the Kennedys, Marcello once admitted to an FBI informant that "yeah I had the little son of a bitch killed, and I would do it again, he was a thorn in my side, I wish I could have done it myself." The same informant reported that Marcello knew Jack Ruby and had also met Lee Harvey Oswald through Marcello's pilot, David Ferrie.

Jack Ruby worked for Joe Civello, Marcello's representative in Dallas, and was active in Marcello's heroin distribution network. Ruby stripper Rose Cheramie was involved in transporting heroin for Ruby at the time of her injury and confinement to a hospital in Eunice, Louisiana, just prior to the assassination (Appendix III).

Marcello's primary source of heroin was the "French Connection" crime syndicate in France. The flow of heroin for the "French Connection" originated in the interior of Indochina and ran through Saigon to laboratories in Marseille, and then on to the large retail markets of the United States. By 1963 heroin trafficking was the most lucrative criminal activity in the U.S., and it generated a massive flow of cash into the coffers of the Mafia, particularly those of Carlos Marcello. [2]

All of this would end with Kennedy's anticipated withdrawal from Vietnam and the subsequent destabilization of the country. The vast profits flowing from "French Connection" heroin were about to disappear with a continued Kennedy Presidency, and this potential loss created a strong economic incentive for some to want to see him dead. It is probably no coincidence that in his deathbed confession former CIA agent E. Howard Hunt described the grassy knoll shooter as a "French Gunman" (Chapter 8).

Fourth, Lyndon Johnson did everything possible to hinder an objective examination of the President's murder. Immediately after the assassination Johnson ordered the Presidential limousine shipped back to Detroit for a complete refurbishing, eliminating all traces of forensic evidence. His aide Cliff Carter had Governor Connally's clothes sent off for cleaning, although it was rather improbable that the Governor would again wear clothes that were full of bullet holes. Johnson formed the Warren Commission with the express purpose of thwarting congressional investigations into the assassination. Johnson issued Executive Order 11652, ensuring that the bulk of assassination evidence would be locked away in the National Archives until 2039. Johnson also confided to his mistress that he knew about the assassination in advance.

Fifth, Lyndon Johnson had a reputation for sexually extreme conduct and his long association and close friendships with Walter Jenkins and J. Edgar Hoover suggest the presence of a network of sexually extreme individuals at the upper echelons of American government. J. Edgar Hoover was a longtime friend of Major Louis Mortimer Bloomfield, the primary shareholder in Permindex, the Swiss corporation linked to assassination attempts on French President Charles de Gaulle. The path of the assassination from the trigger finger of Johnson to the trigger finger of Oswald runs through six homosexuals: Walter Jenkins, J. Edgar Hoover, Clay Shaw, David Ferrie, Jack Ruby, and Lee Harvey Oswald. If allegations that Major Bloomfield was homosexual are true, he would be the seventh in a path that arcs directly from Johnson through Permindex to Oswald.

Homosexuality appears to be a prominent behavioral trait shared by those who organized the Permindex arm of the assassination and by those who executed it.

While Jim Garrison's initial belief that the assassination was a "homosexual thrill killing" is likely not true, it does seem probable that the homosexual underworld was used as a path for the recruitment, motivation, and positioning of Lee Harvey Oswald with a loaded rifle in the sixth floor sniper's nest. One cannot discount the possibility that Hoover may have actively engaged in the strategic sexual blackmail of those involved as a motivational tool to ensure compliance.

Sixth, high ranking CIA agent E. Howard Hunt was photographed in Dealey Plaza after being apprehended in the train yard behind the grassy knoll. Hunt subsequently gave a deathbed confession to his participation and named Lyndon Johnson as the author of the assassination, and several prominent CIA agents as participants.

This implies that in addition to the Permindex-connected conspiracy uncovered by Garrison there may have been other completely different schemes to place additional shooters in Dealey Plaza. E. Howard Hunt's deathbed confession names only prominent CIA employees as participants in the effort to position a "French Gunman" behind the grassy knoll. Marita Lorenz' House Select Committee testimony indicated that a team of CIA trained Operation 40 assassins, including an Oswald double, was sent to Dallas just prior to the assassination. Neither of these scenarios includes Jenkins, Hoover, Bloomfield, Shaw, Ferrie, Ruby, Oswald, or Permindex. A reasonable interpretation is that there were actually three separate and parallel plots that placed three or more shooters in Dealey Plaza, each with little or no direct knowledge of the other.* Of these, only Oswald, the apparent World Communist sympathizer, was destined for discovery and blame.

Seventh, analysis of the acoustical data from the Dallas Police Department indicates with certainty that there was more than one shooter. The data analysis performed by Professors Weiss and Aschkenasy for the House Select Committee on Assassinations found that the trigger pull times

---

* It should be noted, however, that the best opportunity for the sixth floor sniper to shoot the President occurred while the President was slowly headed toward the Texas School Book Depository on Houston Street, before the limousine slowed to make the hairpin turn onto Elm Street, directly underneath the depository. At that point the sniper had a clear shot at the President's entire upper body as it slowly moved towards him at close range. After the first shot the sniper would have had the opportunity for a superior second shot because the limousine would have continued moving towards him with very little opportunity for the President to take cover. The fact that the sixth floor sniper did not fire while the President was slowly coming towards him implies that he had knowledge of the other gunmen and had been instructed to wait until the President was in a triangulated kill zone before firing.

for the last two shots were at 7.49 and 8.31 seconds, only 0.82 seconds apart, and too close together to have been generated by a single shooter using a bolt action rifle.

Regardless of their origin, two shots 0.82 seconds apart indicates a conspiracy. They could not have been fired by the same individual using a bolt action rifle. Further analysis of the original Bolt, Beranek, and Newman data shows that the first shot to hit the President struck him in the back, causing a spinal reflex that brought his tightly bunched fists up to his face. The next shot struck him at the base of his skull, killing him instantly. The third shot to strike the President, fired from the front right, removed the upper right quadrant of his skull and rocketed him back and to the left.

Despite the obvious medical evidence to the contrary, the Warren Commission, the Clark Panel, and the House Select Committee on Assassinations all created an elaborate web of obvious and outrageous lies to disguise the fact that the President had been struck by more than two bullets.

Many date the genesis of the Kennedy assassination to the Bay of Pigs debacle, but in all likelihood it had its origins earlier, in an era when McCarthyism ran rampant in America, and the word of J. Edgar Hoover was enough to ruin one's reputation and life. Hoover hated the Kennedys intensely. If behind the scenes he could intimidate the President through sexual blackmail, he was certainly not above starting rumors of Kennedy's disloyalty to the United States. If the Kennedy Presidency continued past the November 1964 election, he would be fired. Once the assassination plot was hatched it is not difficult to imagine the Director quietly letting it be known, in so many words, that he possessed secret files showing that Kennedy was the dupe of Communists and a security risk, and therefore had to be removed from office for the good of America.

After the disloyalty rumor was rolled like a snowball down a hill, it would eventually become an anti-Communist freight train at the bottom. The pretext would thus be manufactured to assuage anyone with a conscience that they were, in fact, doing the right thing for America by removing Kennedy from office, and from no less an authority figure than J. Edgar Hoover.

Once it is understood that the assassination emanated largely from within the federal government, its outlines become clear. Johnson and Hoover were both astute political observers who used the pockets of intense hatred against the Kennedys to their advantage like pieces on a chessboard. Elements within the Mafia were more than willing to provide killing expertise and funding. Elements within the CIA were more than willing to provide organizational expertise for black operations. Elements within the Secret Service were more than willing to let down the Presidential guard, and assist in destroying and manipulating evidence afterwards. Hoover's counter-intelligence agents in Permindex, L.M. Bloomfield and Clay Shaw, were more than willing to set up the fall guy.

After the assassination, Johnson and Hoover were in complete control of the investigation and they succeeded in keeping one critical fact from ever being officially acknowledged: the President was hit by more than two bullets, and it was therefore impossible that Lee Harvey Oswald acted alone.

If President Kennedy's murder was the crime of the century, then its formal investigation has been the sham of the century, aided and abetted by a complacent and compliant media willing to go along with the Seven Big Lies. And therein lies the real story of who actually killed the President, namely the conduct of those who publicly executed the President and those who covered up, and continue to cover up, this most hideous and horrid crime.

There could, of course, have been a much larger agenda at work in the assassination. Kennedy's playboy ways aside, his views were very much those of an Irish Catholic. His obvious love of family life, his efforts to promote equality for blacks, and his distaste for the use of military brutality as the solution to America's problems were all rooted in his Irish Catholic upbringing. It may well be that Lyndon Johnson, J. Edgar Hoover, and their gang of psychopaths within the federal government simply felt that Catholics like Kennedy didn't fit in with their worldview and plans for the future of America.

APPENDIX I

THE AUTOPSY REPORT

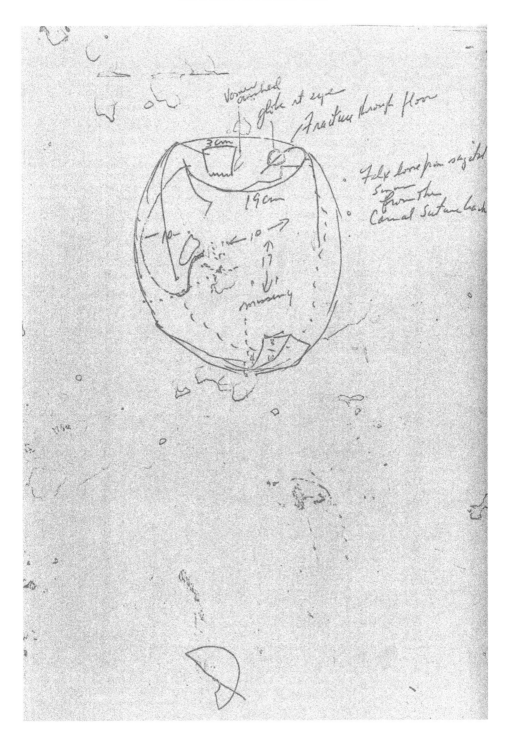

Commission Exhibit No. 387

Standard Form 503
Revised August 1954
Prescribed by
By Bureau of the Budget
Circular A—32 (Rev.)

CLINICAL RECORD				AUTOPSY PROTOCOL	A63-272 (JJB:ec)		
DATE AND HOUR DIED		A. M.	DATE AND HOUR AUTOPSY PERFORMED	A. M.	CHECK ONE		
					FULL AUTOPSY	HEAD ONLY	TRUNK ONLY
22 November 1963 1300(CST)		P. M.	22 November 1963 2000(EST)	M.			
PROSECTOR (497831)			ASSISTANT (439875)		X		
CDR J. J. HUMES, MC, USN			CDR "J" THORNTON BOSWELL,MC,USN				

CLINICAL DIAGNOSES (including operations)   LCOL PIERRE A. FINCK,MC,USA (04 043 322)

Ht. - 72½ inches
Wt. - 170 pounds
Eyes - blue
Hair - Reddish brown

PATHOLOGICAL DIAGNOSES

CAUSE OF DEATH: Gunshot wound, head.

APPROVED SIGNATURE

J. J. HUMES, CDR, MC, USN

MILITARY ORGANIZATION (Base hospital)	AGE	SEX	RACE	IDENTIFICATION NO.	AUTOPSY NO.
PRESIDENT, UNITED STATES	46	Male	Cauc.		A63-272

PATIENT'S IDENTIFICATION (For typed or written entries give: Name—last, first, middle; grade; date; hospital or medical facility)

REGISTER NO.   WARD NO.

KENNEDY, JOHN F.
NAVAL MEDICAL SCHOOL

AUTOPSY PROTOCOL
Standard Form 503

PATHOLOGICAL EXAMINATION REPORT   A63-272   Page 2

CLINICAL SUMMARY: According to available information the
                                                    deceased, President John F. Kennedy,
was riding in an open car in a motorcade during an official visit to Dallas, Texas
on 22 November 1963. The President was sitting in the right rear seat with Mrs.
Kennedy seated on the same seat to his left. Sitting directly in front of the
President was Governor John B. Connolly of Texas and directly in front of Mrs. Kennedy
sat Mrs. Connolly. The vehicle was moving at a slow rate of speed down an incline
into an underpass that leads to a freeway route to the Dallas Trade Mart wherethhe
President was to deliver an address.

                                                    Three shots were heard and the President
fell forward bleeding from the head. (Governor Connolly was seriously wounded by the
same gunfire.) According to newspaper reports ("Washington Post" November 23, 1963)
Bob Jackson, a Dallas "Times Herald"Photographer, said he looked around as he heard
the shots and saw a rifle barrel disappearing into a window on an upper floor of the
nearby Texas School Book Depository Building.

                                                    Shortly following the wounding of the two
men the car was driven to Parkland Hospital in Dallas. In the emergency room of that
hospital the President was attended by Dr. Malcolm Perry. Telephone communication with
Dr. Perry on November 23, 1963 develops the following information relative to the observations made by Dr. Perry and procedures performed there prior to death.

                                                    Dr. Perry noted the massive wound of the
head and a second much smaller wound of the low anterior neck in approximately the
midline. A tracheostomy was performed by extending the latter wound. At this point
bloody air was noted bubbling from the wound and an injury to the right lateral wall
of the trachea was observed. Incisions were made in the upper anterior chest wall
bilaterally to combat possible subcutaneous emphysema. Intravenous infusions of blood
and saline were begun and oxygen was administered. Despite these measures cardiac
arrest occurred and closed chest cardiac massage failed to re-establish cardiac action.
The President was pronounced dead approximately thirty to forty minutes after receiving
his wounds.

                                                    The remains were transported via the
Presidential plane to Washington, D.C. and subsequently to the Naval Medical School,
National Naval Medical Center, Bethesda, Maryland for postmortem examination.

GENERAL DESCRIPTION OF BODY: The body is that of a muscular, well-
                                                    developed and well nourished adult Caucasian
male measuring 72½ inches and weighing approximately 170 pounds. There is beginning
rigor mortis, minimal dependent livor mortis of the dorsum, and early algor mortis. The
hair is reddish brown and abundant, the eyes are blue, the right pupil measuring 8 mm.
in diameter, the left 4 mm. There is edema and ecchymosis of the inner canthus region
of the left eyelid measuring approximately 1.5 cm. in greatest diameter. There is edema
and ecchymosis diffusely over the right supra-orbital ridge with abnormal mobility of
the underlying bone. (The remainder of the scalp will be described with the skull.)

There is clotted blood on the external ears but otherwise the ears, nares, and mouth are essentially unremarkable. The teeth are in excellent repair and there is some pallor of the oral mucous membrane.

Situated on the upper right posterior thorax just above the upper border of the scapula there is a 7 x 4 millimeter oval wound. This wound is measured to be 14 cm. from the tip of the right acromion process and 14 cm. below the tip of the right mastoid process.

Situated in the low anterior neck at approximately the level of the third and fourth tracheal rings is a 6.5 cm. long transverse wound with widely gaping irregular edges. (The depth and character of these wounds wil be further described below.)

Situated on the anterior chest wall in the nipple line are bilateral 2 cm. long recent transverse surgical incisions into the subcutaneous tissue. The one on the left is situated 11 cm. cephalad to the nipple and the one on the right 8 cm. cephalad to the nipple. There is no hemorrhage or ecchymosis associated with these wounds. A similar clean wound measuring 2 cm. in length is situated on the antero-lateral aspect of the left mid arm. Situated on the antero-lateral aspect of each ankle is a recent 2 cm. transverse incision into the subcutaneous tissue.

There is an old well healed 8 cm. McBurney abdominal incision. Over the lumbar spine in the midline is an old, well healed 15 cm. scar. Situated on the upper antero-lateral aspect of the right thigh is an old, well healed 8 cm. scar.

MISSILE WOUNDS: 1. There is a large irregular defect of the scalp and skull on the right involving chiefly the parietal bone but extending somewhat into the temporal and occipital regions. In this region there is an actual absence of scalp and bone producing a defect which measures approximately 13 cm. in greatest diameter.

From the irregular margins of the above scalp defect tears extend in stellate fashion into the more or less intact scalp as follows:

   a. From the right inferior temporo-parietal margin anterior to the right ear to a point slightly above the tragus.

   b. From the anterior parietal margin anteriorly on the forehead to approximately 4 cm. above the right orbital ridge.

   c. From the left margin of the main defect across the midline antero-laterally for a distance of approximately 8 cm.

   d. From the same starting point as c, 10 cm. postero-laterally.

PATHOLOGICAL EXAMINATION REPORT   A63-272   Page 4

Situated in the posterior scalp approximately 2.5 cm. laterally to the right and
slightly above the external occipital protuberance is a lacerated wound measuring
15 x 6 mm. In the underlying bone is a corresponding wound through the skull which
exhibits beveling of the margins of the bone when viewed from the inner aspect of
the skull.

Clearly visible in the above described
large skull defect and exuding from it is lacerated brain tissue which on close
inspection proves to represent the major portion of the right cerebral hemisphere.
At this point it is noted that the falx cerebri is extensively lacerated with disruption of the superior saggital sinus.

Upon reflecting the scalp multiple complete
fracture lines are seen to radiate from both the large defect at the vertex and the
smaller wound at the occiput. These vary greatly in length and direction, the longest
measuring approximately 19 cm. These result in the production of numerous fragments
which vary in size from a few millimeters to 10 cm. in greatest diameter.

The complexity of these fractures and the
fragments thus produced tax satisfactory verbal description and are better appreciated
in photographs and roentgenograms which are prepared.

The brain is removed and preserved for
further study following formalin fixation.

Received as separate specimens from Dallas,
Texas are three fragments of skull bone which in aggregate roughly approximate the
dimensions of the large defect described above. At one angle of the largest of these
fragments is a portion of the perimeter of a roughly circular wound presumably of
exit which exhibits beveling of the outer aspect of the bone and is estimated to
measure approximately 2.5 to 3.0 cm. in diameter. Roentgenograms of this fragment
reveal minute particles of metal in the bone at this margin. Roentgenograms of the
skull reveal multiple minute metallic fragments along a line corresponding with a line
joining the above described small occipital wound and the right supra-orbital ridge.
From the surface of the disrupted right cerebral cortex two small irregularly shaped
fragments of metal are recovered. These measure 7 x 2 mm. and 3 x 1 mm. These are
placed in the custody of Agents Francis X. O'Neill, Jr. and James W. Sibert, of the
Federal Bureau of Investigation, who executed a receipt therefor (attached).

2. The second wound presumably of entry
is that described above in the upper right posterior thorax. Beneath the skin there
is ecchymosis of subcutaneous tissue and musculature. The missile path through the
fascia and musculature cannot be easily probed. The wound presumably of exit was
that described by Dr. Malcolm Parry of Dallas in the low anterior cervical region.
When observed by Dr. Perry the wound measured "a few millimeters in diameter", however it was extended as a tracheostomy incision and thus its character is distorted
at the time of autopsy. However, there is considerable ecchymosis of the strap
muscles of the right side of the neck and of the fascia about the trachea adjacent
to the line of the tracheostomy wound. The third point of reference in connecting

these two wounds is in the apex (supra-clavicular portion) of the right pleural cavity. In this region there is contusion of the parietal pleura and of the extreme apical portion of the right upper lobe of the lung. In both instances the diameter of contusion and ecchymosis at the point of maximal involvement measures 5 cm. Both the visceral and parietal pleura are intact overlying these areas of trauma.

INCISIONS: The scalp wounds are extended in the coronal plane to examine the cranial content and the customary (Y) shaped incision is used to examine the body cavities.

THORACIC CAVITY: The bony cage is unremarkable. The thoracic organs are in their normal positions and relationships and there is no increase in free pleural fluid. The above described area of contusion in the apical portion of the right pleural cavity is noted.

LUNGS: The lungs are of essentially similar appearance the right weighing 320 Gm., the left 290 Gm. The lungs are well aerated with smooth glistening pleural surfaces and gray-pink color. A 5 cm. diameter area of purplish red discoloration and increased firmness to palpation is situated in the apical portion of the right upper lobe. This corresponds to the similar area described in the overlying parietal pleura. Incision in this region reveals recent hemorrhage into pulmonary parenchyma.

HEART: The pericardial cavity is smooth walled and contains approximately 10 cc. of straw-colored fluid. The heart is of essentially normal external contour and weighs 350 Gm. The pulmonary artery is opened in situ and no abnormalities are noted. The cardiac chambers contain moderate amounts of postmortem clotted blood. There are no gross abnormalities of the leaflets of any of the cardiac valves. The following are the circumferences of the cardiac valves: aortic 7.5 cm., pulmonic 7 cm., tricuspid 12 cm., mitral 11 cm. The myocardium is firm and reddish brown. The left ventricular myocardium averages 1.2 cm. in thickness, the right ventricular myocardium 0.4 cm. The coronary arteries are dissected and are of normal distribution and smooth walled and elastic throughout.

ABDOMINAL CAVITY: The abdominal organs are in their normal positions and relationships and there is no increase in free peritoneal fluid. The vermiform appendix is surgically absent and there are a few adhesions joining the region of the cecum to the ventral abdominal wall at the above described old abdominal incisional scar.

SKELETAL SYSTEM: Aside from the above described skull wounds there are no significant gross skeletal abnormalities.

PHOTOGRAPHY: Black and white and color photographs depicting significant findings are exposed but not developed. These photographs were placed in the custody of Agent Roy H. Kellerman of the U. S. Secret Service, who executed a receipt therefore (attached).

PATHOLOGICAL EXAMINATION REPORT   A63-272   Page 6

ROENTGENOGRAMS: Roentgenograms are made of the entire body and of the separately submitted three fragments of skull bone. These are developed and were placed in the custody of Agent Roy H. Kellerman of the U. S. Secret Service, who executed a receipt therefor (attached).

SUMMARY: Based on the above observations it is our opinion that the deceased died as a result of two perforating gunshot wounds inflicted by high velocity projectiles fired by a person or persons unknown. The projectiles were fired from a point behind and somewhat above the level of the deceased. The observations and available information do not permit a satisfactory estimate as to the sequence of the two wounds.

     The fatal missile entered the skull above and to the right of the external occipital protuberance. A portion of the projectile traversed the cranial cavity in a posterior-anterior direction (see lateral skull roentgenograms) depositing minute particles along its path. A portion of the projectile made its exit through the parietal bone on the right carrying with it portions of cerebrum, skull and scalp. The two wounds of the skull combined with the force of the missile produced extensive fragmentation of the skull, laceration of the superior saggital sinus, and of the right cerebral hemisphere.

     The other missile entered the right superior posterior thorax above the scapula and traversed the soft tissues of the supra-scapular and the supra-clavicular portions of the base of the right side of the neck. This missile produced contusions of the right apical parietal pleura and of the apical portion of the right upper lobe of the lung. The missile contused the strap muscles of the right side of the neck, damaged the trachea and made its exit through the anterior surface of the neck. As far as can be ascertained this missile struck no bony structures in its path through the body.

     In addition, it is our opinion that the wound of the skull produced such extensive damage to the brain as to preclude the possibility of the deceased surviving this injury.

     A supplementary report will be submitted following more detailed examination of the brain and of microscopic sections. However, it is not anticipated that these examinations will materially alter the findings.

J. J. HUMES
CDR, MC, USN (497831)

THORNTON BOSWELL
CDR, MC, USN (489878)

PIERRE A. FINCK
LT COL, MC, USA
(04-043-322)

APPENDIX II

BLAKEY MEMORANDUM CONCERNING THE ACOUSTICAL ANALYSIS

TO: All Select Committee Members

FROM: G. Robert Blakey, Chief Counsel and Director

DATE: February 22, 1979

RE: Fine Points of Correlation of Tape to Film

        As noted during the course of our public hearings, any attempt
to derive the maximum knowledge from the available acoustical and
photographic evidence requires that at least an approximate correlation be made between the timing of the shots as recorded on the
Dallas Police Department tape and the visual record contained in the
Zapruder film. One such correlation was presented during the hearings in the form of a copy of the Zapruder film with four shots dubbed onto it at the approximate times that the occupants of the
limousine would have heard the sounds of the gun fire. In fact, two
different versions of the film were shown on December 29th. In the
first, the sound of the fourth shot (from the TSBD) coincided with
the fatal head wound seen at Zapruder frame 313, and in the second,
the third (grassy knoll shot) coincided with that wound.

        Under the time constraints of preparing for the hearings on
December 29th and with the recognition that neither the running
speed of the DPD dictabelt nor of Zapruder's camera was known with
absolute precision, the frames used on December 29th for such
correlation purposes were based only on the actual spacing of shots
on the DPD tape (totaling 7.9 seconds from the first to the last) and
the "average" running speed of Zapruder's camera, which the FBI
determined in 1964 to be 18.3 frames per second.

        Nevertheless, so that the Committee's final report may be more
exact and that you can understand the basis for the increased precision we have continued to refine our data and it may be helpful to
note in this memorandum the results of our efforts to be more precise
as well as what is set forth in the final reports of DB&N, Weiss and
Aschkenasy, and what was contained in a letter from FBI Director
Hoover to the Warren Commission of February 3, 1964.

        In its final report, BB&N advises the Committee that its best
estimate is that the DPD dictabelt was recording approximately 5%
too slowly on November 22, 1963, a fact also noted in the hearing
on the 29th. The FBI's letter of February 3, 1964, also stated as
quoted in full below:

            At the request of members of your staff the FBI
        Laboratory has made a further study of the film speed
        of the camera used by Mr. Abraham Zapruder in filming the
        eight millimeter motion picture of the President's
        assassination. You have previously been furnished the
        results of the Laboratory examination of this camera
        which places the film speed at 18 1/3 frames per second.
        The Laboratory was requested to establish, if possible,
        the variation between the film speed of the camera
        when the drive spring is fully wound and when the spring
        is almost run down.

            This study has been made by checking the film
        speed of the Zapruder camera at ten second intervals
        throughout the full running time of a fully wound camera.
        Several checks were made on a full roll of film and it
        was found that the film speed of the camera when fully
        wound runs at an average speed of from 18.0 to 18.1 frames

2 - correlation of tape to film

per second (fps) for the first ten seconds. It gradually
increases to 18.3 to 18.5 fps for the next twenty seconds,
then gradually decreases slightly to 18.1 fps for ten
seconds before the final twenty seconds that run at an
average speed of 17.6 to 17.9 frames per second. Mr.
Zapruder has stated that the camera was fully wound when
he started filming the President's motorcade. Since all
of Mr. Zapruder's assassination film was exposed well
within the first half of time the camera will run on one
winding, the rundown film speed should not be considered
in the calculations. Therefore, the above figures result
in our previous average frames per second speed for the
assassination film of 18 1/3 or 18.3 frames per second.

Shots 1, 2 and 4 were found by BB&N to begin on the DPD tape
at 137.70, 139.27 and 145.61 seconds, respectively. Shot number
three was found by Weiss and Aschkenasy to begin at 144.90 seconds.
If the spacing between those shots is adjusted by the approximate
5% error in running speed of the dictabelt, the probable true
timing of the shots, beginning with shot number one as zero, is
0.0, 1.65, 7.6 and 8.3 seconds.

Using those best estimates of the true timing of the shots,
it is possible to calculate the frame number on Zapruder's film at
which any event of interest occurred, and to do so for any assumed
running speed of the camera. Nevertheless, it would not be accurate
to simply multiply the corrected time spacing of the sounds as recorded, by the assumed number of frames per second running speed,
unless, of course, you wanted to know only what frame was being
exposed when the microphone picked up the sound of each shot.

If, for example, what you wished to know was which frame of
the film was exposed when the bullet struck (or passed by) the
limousine on the first shot, and you assumed the camera was running
at 18.5 frames per second, and that the fatal head wound was caused
by the fourth (TSBD) shot, your calculations would proceed as
follows:

1. The distance from the motorcycle to the TSBD at the time
    of the first shot was approximately 124 feet.

2. Since sound traveled at approximately 1123 fps on 11/22/63
    in Dealey Plaza (it being about 65° in the Plaza at that
    time), the sound took about .11 second to reach the micro-
    phone after the muzzle blast occurred. Stated conversely,
    the trigger was pulled .11 second <u>before</u> the 0.0 point
    in time on the tape.

3. If the fatal head shot is observable at frame 313, we can
    assume the bullet struck one frame earlier, at 312. A
    Mannlicher-Carcano bullet travels at approximately 2000 fps.
    Since the limousine was approximately 265 feet from the
    TSBD window at frame 312, the trigger was pulled .13
    seconds before frame 312. ($\frac{265}{2000}$ = .13) The motorcycle
    was only about 145 feet from the TSBD at this time.
    Consequently, dividing 145 by 1123, it is apparent that
    the microphone recorded that sound .13 seconds after the
    trigger pull, or at about the same time that the bullet
    impacted.

4. It is now possible to determine the frame at which the
    trigger pull on shot number one occurred. You simply take
    the total corrected tape time (8.3 seconds), add the

229

3 - correlation of tape to film

.11 second delay from shot number one trigger pull to recording time (step numer 2), multiply by 18.5 frames per second (8.41 x 18.5 = 155.6), and substract from 312. The trigger was first pulled at frame 156.

5. Finally, by allowing for bullet travel time to the limousine (about 143 feet), it can be determined that the bullet struck at about frame 157 (156 + ($\frac{143}{2000}$ x 18.5) = 157).

Similar calculations can be made for other events of interest. One example is the question of what frame was being exposed when Zapruder heard each shot. This information, of course, is useful for comparison with the blur analysis conducted by the photographic panel.

The following is a chart setting forth the results of such calculations, using three different estimates of camera speed, 18.0, 18.3, and 18.5 frames per seconds:

Shot No.	Tape Time	Trigger Pull Time	Hearing Shock Wave in Limo.		Hearing Muzzle Blast by Zapruder[3]		Weapon to Limo.[2]	Motorcycle to Weapon[1]
1	0.11	0		161 177		165 181		
			0.07	159 175	0.24	162 178	143'	124'
				157 173		160 177		
2	1.76	1.66		191 208		194 210		
			1.74	189 206	1.90	192 209	165'	107'
				188 205		191 208		
3	7.69	7.49		296 312		296 312		
			7.55	296 312	7.55	296 312	111'	220'
				295 312		295 312		
4	8.44	8.31		312 328		314 330		
			8.44	312 328	8.55	314 330	266'	144'
				312 329		314 330		

[1] Sound: 1123 fps
[2] Bullet: 2000 fps

[3] Zapruder to TSBD: 270'
Zapruder to Knoll: 60'

APPENDIX III

THE ACCOUNT OF ROSE CHERAMIE

ROSE CHERAMIE

(1)   According to accounts of assassinations researchers, a woman known as Rose Cheramie, a heroin addict and prostitute with a long history of arrests, was found on November 20, 1963, lying on the road near Eunice, La., bruised and disoriented.(*1*) She was taken to the Louisiana State Hospital in Jackson, La., to recover from her injuries and what appeared to be narcotics withdrawal.(*2*) Cheramie reportedly told the attending physician that President Kennedy was going to be killed during his forthcoming visit to Dallas.(*3*) The doctor did not pay much attention to the ravings of a patient going "cold turkey" until after the President was assassinated 2 days later.(*4*) State police were called in and Cheramie was questioned at length.(*5*) She reportedly told police officers she had been a stripper in Jack Ruby's night club and was transporting a quantity of heroin from Florida to Houston at Ruby's insistence when she quarreled with two men also participating in the dope run.(*6*) Cheramie said the men pushed her out of a moving vehicle and left her for dead.(*7*) After the assassination, Cheramie maintained Ruby and Lee Harvey Oswald had known each other well.(*8*) She said she had seen Oswald at Ruby's night club and claimed Oswald and Ruby had been homosexual partners.(*9*)

(2)   Ironically, the circumstances of Rose Cheramie's death are strikingly similar to the circumstances surrounding her original involvement in the assassination investigation. Cheramie died of injuries received from an automobile accident on a strip of highway near Big Sandy, Tex., in the early morning of September 4, 1965.(*10*) The driver stated Cheramie had been lying in the roadway and although he attempted to avoid hitting her, he ran over the top of her skull, causing fatal injuries.(*11*) An investigation into the accident and the possibility of a relationship between the victim and the driver produced no evidence of foul play.(*12*) The case was closed.(*13*)

(3)   Although Cheramie's allegations were eventually discounted, her death 2 years later prompted renewed speculation about her story. It was noted, for example, that over 50 individuals who had been associated with the investigation of the Kennedy assassination had died within 3 years of that event.(*14*) The deaths, by natural or other causes, were labeled "mysterious" by Warren Commission critics and the news media.(*15*) The skeptics claim that the laws of probability would show the number of deaths is so unlikely as to be highly suspect.(*16*) As detailed elsewhere, the committee studied such claims and determined they were erroneous.(*17*) Nevertheless, allegations involving Rose Cheramie, often counted among the "mysterious" deaths, was of particular interest to the committee, since it indicated a possible association of Lee Harvey Oswald and Jack Ruby: an association of these individuals with members of organized crime; and possible connection between Cheramie's confinement at the State Hospital in Jackson, La.

(199)

232

and Oswald's search for employment there in the summer of 1963.
(4)   The committee set out to obtain a full account of the Cheramie allegations and determine whether her statements could be at all corroborated. The committee interviewed and deposed pertinent witnesses. Files from U.S. Customs and the FBI were requested. Information developed during the investigation by New Orleans District Attorney Jim Garrison was examined. Records of Cheramie's hospitalization at the East Louisiana State Hospital were studied.
(5)   Hospital records indicate Melba Christine Marcades, alias Rose Cheramie, was brought to the State Hospital in Jackson, La. by police from Eunice on November 21, 1963 and officially admitted at 6 a.m.(*18*) She was originally from Houston, Tex., where her mother still lived. (*19*) She was approximately 34 years old in 1963, had used many aliases throughout her lifetime and had lived many years in Louisiana and Texas.(*20*)
(6)   According to the clinical notes, the deputy accompanying Cheramie said the patient had been "picked up on [the] side of [the] road and had been given something by the coroner."(*21*) The coroner in Eunice was contacted by doctors at the hospital and he told them Cheramie had been coherent when he spoke with her at 10:30 p.m., November 20, but he did administer a sedative.(*22*) He further indicated that Cheramie was a 9-year mainlining heroin addict, whose last injection had been around 2 p.m., November 20.(*23*) The doctors noted that Cheramie's condition upon initial examination indicated heroin withdrawal and clinical shock.(*24*)
(7)– Relevant to Cheramie's credibility was an assessment of her mental state. From November 22 to November 24, Cheramie required close attention and medication.(*25*) On November 25 she was transferred to the ward.(*26*) On November 27 she was released to Louisiana State Police Lieutenant Fruge.(*27*)
(8)   The hospital records gave no reference as to alleged statements made by Cheramie or why she was released to Lieutenant Fruge on November 27, 1963. These records do indicate Cheramie had been hospitalized for alcoholism and narcotics addiction on other occasions, including commitment to the same hospital in March 1961 by the criminal court of New Orleans.(*28*) During this stay, the woman was diagnosed as ". . . without psychosis. However, because of her previous record of drug addiction she may have a mild integrative and pleasure defect."(*29*) Her record would show she has "intervals of very good behavior" but at other times she "presents episodically psychopathic behavior" indicative in her history of drug and alcohol abuse, prostitution, arrest on numerous, if minor, charges.(*30*)
(9)   The committee interviewed one of the doctors on staff at East Louisiana State Hospital who had seen Cheramie during her stay there at the time of the Kennedy assassination.(*31*) The doctor corroborated aspects of the Cheramie allegations. Dr. Victor Weiss verified that he was employed as a resident physician at the hospital in 1963.(*32*) He recalled that on Monday, November 25, 1963, he was asked by another physician, Dr. Bowers, to see a patient who had been committed November 20 or 21.(*33*) Dr. Bowers allegedly told Weiss that the patient, Rose Cheramie, had stated before the assassination that President Kennedy was going to be killed.(*34*) Weiss questioned Cheramie about

her statements.(*35*) She told him she had worked for Jack Ruby. She did not have any specific details of a particular assassination plot against Kennedy, but had stated the "word in the underworld" was that Kennedy would be assassinated.(*36*) She further stated that she had been traveling from Florida to her home in Texas when the man traveling with her threw her from the automobile in which they were riding.(*37*)

(10) Francis Fruge, a lieutenant with the Louisiana State Police in 1963, was the police officer who first came to Cheramie's assistance on November 20, 1963, had her committed to the State Hospital, and later released her into his custody following the assassination to investigate her allegations.(*38*) As such, he provided an account further detailing her allegations and the official response to her allegations.

(11) Fruge was deposed by the committee on April 18, 1978. (*39*) He told the committee he was called on November 20, 1963 by an administrator at a private hospital in Eunice, La. that a female accident victim had been taken there for treatment.(*40*) She had been treated for minor abrasions, and although she appeared to be under the influence of drugs since she had "no financial basis" she was to be released.(*41*) Fruge did what he normally did in such instances. As the woman required no further medical attention, he put her in a jail cell to sober up.(*42*) This arrangement did not last long. The woman began to display severe symptoms of withdrawal.(*43*) Fruge said he called a doctor, who sedated Cheramie and Fruge transported Cheramie to the State hospital in Jackson, La.(*44*)

(12) Fruge said that during the "1 to 2 hour" ride to Jackson, he asked Cheramie some "routine" questions.(*45*) Fruge told the committee:

> She related to me that she was coming from Florida to Dallas with two men who were Italians or resembled Italians. They had stopped at this lounge . . . and they'd had a few drinks and had gotten into an argument or something. The manager of the lounge threw her out and she got on the road and hitchhiked to catch a ride, and this is when she got hit by a vehicle.(*46*)

Fruge said the lounge was a house of prostitution called the Silver Slipper.(*47*) Fruge asked Cheramie what she was going to do in Dallas: "She said she was going to, number one, pick up some money, pick up her baby, and to kill Kennedy."(*48*) Fruge claimed during these intervals that Cheramie related the story she appeared to be quite lucid. (*49*) Fruge had Cheramie admitted to the hospital late on November 20.(*50*)

(13) On November 22, when he heard the President had been assassinated, Fruge said he immediately called the hospital and told them not to release Cheramie until he had spoken to her.(*51*) The hospital administrators assented but said Fruge would have to wait until the following Monday before Cheramie would be well enough to speak to anyone.(*52*) Fruge waited. Under questioning, Cheramie told Fruge that the two men traveling with her from Miami were going to Dallas to kill the President.(*53*) For her part, Cheramie was to obtain $8,000 from an unidentified source in Dallas and proceed to Houston with the two men to complete a drug deal.(*54*) Cheramie was also supposed to

202

pick up her little boy from friends who had been looking after him.(*55*)
(14)   Cheramie further supplied detailed accounts of the arrangement for the drug transaction in Houston.(*56*) She said reservations
had been made at the Rice Hotel in Houston.(*57*) The trio was to meet
a seaman who was bringing in 8 kilos of heroin to Galveston by
boat.(*58*) Cheramie had the name of the seaman and the boat he
was arriving on.(*59*) Once the deal was completed, the trio would
proceed to Mexico.(*60*)
(15) Fruge told the committee that he repeated Cheramie's story to
his supervisors and asked for instructions.(*61*) He was told to follow
up on it.(*62*) Fruge promptly took Cheramie into custody—as indicated in hospital records—and set out to check her story.(*63*) He
contacted the chief customs agent in Galveston who reportedly verified
the scheduled docking of the boat and the name of the seaman.(*64*)
Fruge believed the customs agent was also able to verify the name of
the man in Dallas who was holding Cheramie's son.(*65*) Fruge recalled
that the customs agent had tailed the seaman as he disembarked from
the boat, but then lost the man's trail.(*70*) Customs closed the case.(*71*)
(16)   Fruge had also hoped to corroborate other statements made by
Cheramie. During a flight from Houston, according to Fruge,
Cheramie noticed a newspaper with headlines indicating investigators
had not been able to establish a relationship between Jack Ruby and
Lee Harvey Oswald.(*72*) Cheramie laughed at the headline, Fruge
said.(*73*) Cheramie told him she had worked for Ruby, or "Pinky,"
as she knew him, at his night club in Dallas and claimed Ruby and
Oswald "had been shacking up for years.(*74*) Fruge said he called
Capt. Will Fritz of the Dallas Police Department with this informa-
tion.(*75*) Fritz answered, he wasn't interested.(*76*) Fritz and the
Louisiana State Police dropped the investigation into the matter.(*77*)
(17)   Four years later, however, investigators from the office of
District Attorney Garrison in New Orleans contacted Fruge.(*78*)
Fruge went on detail to Garrison's office to assist in the investigation into the Kennedy assassination.(*79*)
(18)   During the course of the New Orleans D.A.'s investigation
Fruge was able to pursue leads in the Cheramie case that he had not
checked out in the original investigation. Although there appeared
to be different versions as to how Cheramie ended up by the side of
the road, and the number and identity of her companions, Fruge
attempted to corroborate the version she had given him. Fruge spoke
with the owner of the Silver Slipper Lounge.(*80*) The bar owner, a
Mr. Mac Manual since deceased, told Fruge that Cheramie had come
in with two men who the owner knew as pimps engaged in the business
of hauling prostitutes in from Florida.(*81*) When Cheramie became
intoxicated and rowdy, one of the men "slapped her around" and threw
her outside.(*82*)
(19)   Fruge claims that he showed the owner of the bar a "stack" of
photographs and mug shots to identify.(*83*) According to Fruge, the
barowner chose the photos of a Cuban exile, Sergio Arcacha Smith,
and another Cuban Fruge believed to be named Osanto.(*84*) Arcacha
Smith was known to Kennedy assassination investigators as an anti-
Castro Cuban refugee who had been active in 1961 as the head of the
New Orleans Cuban Revolutionary Front.(*85*) At that time, he befriended anti-Castro activist and commercial pilot David Ferrie, who

was named and dismissed as a suspect in the Kennedy assassination within days of the President's death.(*86*) Ferrie and Arcacha Smith were also believed to have had ties with New Orleans organized crime figure Carlos Marcello.(*87*) Arcacha Smith moved from the New Orleans area in 1962 to go to Miami and later to settle in Houston.(*88*) The weekend following the assassination, Ferrie took a trip to Houston and Galveston for a little "rest and relaxation," while police searched New Orleans for him after receiving a tip he had been involved in the assassination.(*89*) The committee has found credible evidence indicating Ferrie and Oswald were seen together in August 1963 in the town of Clinton, La., 13 miles from the hospital in Jackson where Cheramie was treated and where Oswald reportedly sought employment. Allegations regarding Arcacha Smith and Ferrie and the committee's investigation are set forth in detail elsewhere in the Report. (*90*) Clearly, evidence of a link between Cheramie and Arcacha Smith would be highly significant, Arcacha Smith, however, denied any knowledge of Cheramie and her allegations. Other avenues of corroboration of Fruge's identification of Cheramie's traveling companion as Sergio Arcacha Smith and further substantiation of Cheramie's allegations remained elusive.

(20)   U.S. Customs was unable to locate documents and reports related to its involvement in the Cheramie investigation although such involvement was not denied.(*91*) Nor could customs officials locate those agents named by Fruge as having participated in the original investigation, as they had since left the employ of the agency.(*92*)

(21)   Since the FBI had never been notified by the Louisiana State Police and U.S. Customs of their interest in Cheramie, the FBI file did not have any reference to the Cheramie allegations of November 1963.(*93*) FBI files did give reference to the investigation of a tip from Melba Mercades, actually Rose Cheramie, in Ardmore, Okla. that she was en route to Dallas to deliver $2,600 worth of heroin to a man in Oak Cliff, Tex.(*94*) She was then to proceed to Galveston, Tex., to pick up a load of narcotics from a seaman on board a ship destined for Galveston in the next few days.(*95*) She gave "detailed descriptions as to individuals, names, places, and amounts distributed."(*96*) Investigations were conducted by narcotics bureaus in Oklahoma and Texas and her information was found to be "erroneous in all respects."(*97*)

(22)   A similar tale was told in 1965: FBI agents investigated a tip from Rozella Clinkscales, alias Melba Marcades, alias Rose Cheramie.(*98*) Like the stories told in 1963, Cheramie-Clinkscales claimed individuals associated with the syndicate were running prostitution rings in several southern cities such as Houston and Galveston, Tex., Oklahoma City, Okla. and Montgomery, Ala. by transporting hookers, including Cheramie-Clinkscales, from town to town. (*99*) Furthermore, she claimed she had information about a heroin deal operating from a New Orleans ship.(*100*) A call to the Coast Guard verified an ongoing narcotics investigation of the ship.(*101*) Other allegations made by Cheramie-Clinkscales could not be verified. Further investigation into Cheramie-Clinkscales revealed she had apparently previously furnished the FBI false information concerning her involvement in prostitution and narcotics matters and that she had been confined to a mental institution in Norman, Okla. on three

204

occasions. (*102*) FBI agents decided to pursue the case no further. (*103*) The FBI indicated agents did not know of the death of their informant on September 4, 1965, occurring just 1 month after she had contacted the FBI. Louisiana State Police investigating Cheramie's fatal accident also apparently did not know of the FBI's interest in her.

Submitted by,

PATRICIA ORR, *Researcher.*

REFERENCES

(*1*) "The Bizarre Deaths Following JFK's Murder," *Argosy.* March 1977, Vol. 384, No. 8, p. 52 (JFK Document No. 002559).
(*2*) Ibid.
(*3*) Ibid.
(*4*) Ibid.
(*5*) Ibid.
(*6*) Ibid.
(*7*) Ibid.
(*8*) Ibid.
(*9*) Ibid.
(*10*) Louisiana State Police Memo, from Lt. Francis Fruge, Parish of St. Landry, April 4, 1967, in (JFK Document No. 013520).
(*11*) Ibid.
(*12*) Ibid.
(*13*) Ibid.
(*14*) "The Bizarre Deaths . . ." See FN No. 1.
(*15*) Ibid.
(*16*) Ibid.
(*17*) See Anti-Castro Cuban section of the Staff Reports.
(*18*) East Louisiana State Hospital, Jackson, La., records for Melba Christine Marcades AKA Rose Cheramie, (JFK Document No. 006097).
(*19*) Ibid.
(*20*) Ibid. Note: FBI records list Cheramie's (Marcades) birthdate as October 14, 1932, in Dallas, Tex. (See FBI file No. 166-1640 in JFK Document No. 012979).
(*21*) Ibid.
(*22*) Ibid.
(*23*) Ibid.
(*24*) Ibid.
(*25*) Ibid.
(*26*) Ibid.
(*27*) Ibid.
(*28*) Ibid.
(*29*) Ibid.
(*30*) Ibid.
(*31*) HSCA Contact Report, July 5, 1978, Bob Buras (with Dr. Victor Weiss), (JFK Document No. 009609).
(*32*) Ibid.
(*33*) Ibid.
(*34*) Ibid.
(*35*) Ibid.
(*36*) Ibid.
(*37*) Ibid.
(*38*) HSCA Contact Report, April 7, 1978, Bob Buras (with Mr. Francis Louis Fruge), p. 1 (JFK Document No. 014141).
(*39*) HSCA Deposition of Francis Louis Fruge, April 18, 1978 (JFK Document No. 014570).
(*40*) Id. at p. 4-5.
(*41*) Id. at p. 5.
(*42*) Ibid.
(*43*) Id. at p. 6.
(*44*) Ibid.
(*45*) Id. at p. 8.
(*46*) Ibid.
(*47*) Id. at p. 9.

(48) Id. at p. 13.
(49) Ibid.
(50) Ibid.
(51) Id. at p. 12.
(52) Ibid.
(53) Id. at p. 13.
(54) Id. at p. 14.
(55) Ibid.
(56) Ibid.
(57) Ibid.
(58) Ibid.
(59) Ibid.
(60) Ibid.
(61) Ibid.
(62) Id. at p. 15.
(63) Id. at p. 17; East Louisiana State Hospital, Jackson, La., records for Melba Christine Marcades AKA Rose Cheramie (JFK Document No. 006097).
(64) HSCA Deposition of Francis Louis Fruge, April 18, 1978, p. 20 (JFK Document No. 014570).
(65) Id. at p. 22.
(66) Ibid.
(67) Id. at p. 18.
(68) Id. at p. 22.
(69) Id. at p. 23.
(70) Ibid.
(71) Ibid.
(72) Id. at p. 19.
(73) Ibid.
(74) Ibid. Note: Fruge also indicated the Club was called the "Pink Door," although Ruby is not known to have ever had a club by this name. See also, Louisiana State Police Memo., April 4, 1967, from Lt. Francis Fruge, Parish of St. Landry, in JFK Document No. 013520).
(75) Id. at p. 20.
(76) Ibid.
(77) Ibid.
(78) Id. at p. 24.
(79) Id. at p. 25.
(80) Id. at p. 27–8.
(81) Id. at p. 27.
(82) Id. at p. 28. See also HSCA Contact Report, April 7, 1978, Bob Buras (with Francis Louis Fruge) (JFK Document No. 0141414).
(83) Id. at p. 28.
(84) Id. at p. 28, 30.
(85) See Staff Report on Anti-Castro Cuban activity.
(86) Ibid.
(87) Ibid.
(88) Ibid.
(89) See Staff Report on Anti-Castro activity.
(90) Ibid.
(91) See Staff Memo., Rose Cheramie File, contact with Dennis Cronin, U.S. Customs (JFK Document No. 013520).
(92) HSCA Contact Report, June 26, 1978, Marty Daly (with U.S. Customs), (JFK Document No. 009481).
(93) See FBI file No. 166–1604 for Melba Christine Marcades, Vol. 1 of 1, (JFK Document No. 012979).
(94) Id. at FBI 166–1604–3, February 11, 1966, Enclosure No. 1.
(95) Id. at FBI 166–1604–2, December 14, 1965, Enclosure.
(96) Ibid.
(97) Ibid.
(98) Id. at FBI 166–1604–1, November 23, 1965, p. 1.
(99) Id. at p. 3.
(100) Id. at p. 2.
(101) Id. at p. 4.
(102) Ibid.
(103) Ibid.
(104) East Louisana State Hospital, Jackson, La., records for Melba Christine Marcades AKA Rose Cheramie (JFK Document No. 006097).

NOTES

CHAPTER 1

1. History Channel, *JFK: 3 Shots That Changed America*, 1:49:45 – 1:50:30.
2. Warren Commission Report, p. x.
3. Warren Commission Report, p. 3.
4. Warren Commission Report, p. 4.
5. Ibid.
6. Warren Commission Report, p. 5.
7. Warren Commission Report, p. 6.
8. Warren Commission Report, pp. 6 - 7.
9. Warren Commission Report, pp. 8 – 9.
10. Warren Commission Report, pp. 9 – 10.
11. Warren Commission Report, p. 11.
12. Warren Commission Report, pp. 11 – 13.
13. Warren Commission Report, pp. 13 – 14.
14. Warren Commission Report, pp. 14 – 15.
15. Warren Commission Report, p. 15.
16. Ibid.
17. Ibid.
18. Warren Commission Report, p. 16.
19. Warren Commission Report, p. 17.
20. Warren Commission Report, pp. 18 - 25.
21. Warren Commission Hearings and Exhibits, Commission Exhibit 392, Vol. XVII, pp. 2 – 3, 10.
22. Warren Commission Hearings and Exhibits, Commission Exhibit 392, Vol. XVII, pp. 14 – 15.
23. Warren Commission Hearings and Exhibits, Commission Exhibit 392, Vol. XVII, p. 8.
24. Warren Commission Hearings and Exhibits, Commission Exhibit 392, Vol. XVII, p. 6.
25. Warren Commission Hearings and Exhibits, Commission Exhibit 392,

Vol. XVII, p. 5.

26. Warren Commission Hearings and Exhibits, Commission Price Exhibit 21, Vol. XXI, p. 216.
27. Warren Commission Hearings and Exhibits, Vol. II, p. 141.
28. Weisberg, Harold. *John F. Kennedy Assassination Post Mortem*, pp. 531 – 536.
29. Warren Commission Report, p. 89.
30. Warren Commission Hearings and Exhibits, Commission Exhibit 397, Vol. XVII, p. 48.
31. Warren Commission Report, p. 92.
32. Warren Commission Hearings and Exhibits, Commission Exhibit 392, Vol. XVII, p. 14.
33. Garrison, Jim. *On the Trail of the Assassins*, pp. 288 – 292.
34. Warren Commission Report, pp. 96 – 117.
35. Warren Commission Hearings and Exhibits, Vol. II, p. 382.
36. Warren Commission Hearings and Exhibits, Vol. II, p. 375.

CHAPTER 2

1. Probe. *The Formation of the Clark Panel*, Vol. 3, No. 1, 1995.
2. Corson, William, Trento, Susan, and Trento, Joseph. *Widows.*
3. Hougan, Jim. *Secret Agenda.*
4. Clark Panel Report, pp. 1 – 16.
5. Chicago Tribune, January 17, 1969, p. 1.

CHAPTER 3

1. Groden, Robert, and Livingstone, Harrison. *High Treason: The Assassination of President Kennedy - What Really Happened*, pp. 291 – 345.
2. Warren Commission Hearings and Exhibits, Vol. VI, p. 33.
3. Hearings Before the Select Committee on Assassinations, Vol. 1, pp. 141 – 146.

4. Hearings Before the Select Committee on Assassinations, Vol. 1, pp. 238 – 302.
5. Hearings Before the Select Committee on Assassinations, Vol. 1, pp. 301 – 302.
6. Hearings Before the Select Committee on Assassinations, Vol. 1, pp. 332 –374.
7. Hearings Before the Select Committee on Assassinations, Vol. 1, pp. 376 – 379.
8. Hearings Before the Select Committee on Assassinations, Vol. 2, pp. 16 – 17.
9. Hearings Before the Select Committee on Assassinations, Vol. 2, pp. 17 – 106.
10. Thomas, D.B. *Echo Correlation Analysis and the Acoustic Evidence in the Kennedy Assassination Revisited*, Science & Justice, 41(1): 21 – 32.
11. Thomas, Donald. *Hear No Evil: Politics, Science & the Forensic Evidence in the Kennedy Assassination*.
12. Report of the Select Committee on Assassinations of the House of Representatives.

CHAPTER 4

1. Hitler, Adolf. *Mein Kampf*, Vol. I, Ch. X (translated by James Murphy).
2. Warren Commission Report, p. 86.
3. Hearings Before the Select Committee on Assassinations, Vol. 1, p. 329.
4. Thomas, Donald. *Hear No Evil*, p. 288.

CHAPTER 5

1. Warren Commission Report, p. 363.
2. History Channel. *The Men Who Killed Kennedy: The Truth Shall Set You Free*, 17:20 – 28:20.
3. Ventura, Jesse, Russell, Dick, and Wayne, David. *They Killed Our President*, pp. 123 - 128.

CHAPTER 6

1. Posner, Gerald. *Case Closed: Lee Harvey Oswald and the Assassination of JFK*.
2. Bugliosi, Vincent. *Reclaiming History*.
3. O'Reilly, Bill, and Dugard, Martin. *Killing Kennedy: The End of Camelot*.
4. Blakey, G. Robert, and Billings, Richard. *The Plot to Kill the President: Organized Crime Assassinated JFK*.
5. Waldron, Lamar, and Hartmann, Thom. *Ultimate Sacrifice*, pp. 412 - 415.
6. O'Leary, Brad, and Seymour, L.E. *Triangle of Death: The Shocking Truth about the Role of South Vietnam and the French Mafia in the Assassination of JFK*.
7. Stone, Roger. *The Man Who Killed Kennedy: The Case Against LBJ*.
8. Nelson, Phillip. *LBJ: The Mastermind of the JFK Assassination*.

CHAPTER 7

1. Livingstone, Harrison. *High Treason 2, The Great Coverup: The Assassination of President John F. Kennedy*, p. 224.
2. New York Times, November 24, 1963, p. 5.
3. Magoun, H.W. *The Waking Brain*, pp. 74 – 112.
4. House Select Committee on Assassinations Report, Vol. VII, p. 289.
5. Thornburn, William. *Cases of Injury to the Cervical Region of the Spinal Cord*.
6. Lattimer, John. *Kennedy and Lincoln: Medical and Ballistic Comparisons of Their Assassinations*.
7. Warren Commission Report, p. 646.
8. Lane, Mark. *Rush to Judgment*, p. 411.
9. House Select Committee on Assassinations Report, Vol. VII, p. 20.
10. Warren Commission Report, p. 91.
11. House Select Committee on Assassinations Report, Vol. VII, p. 247.
12. Thompson, Josiah. *Six Seconds in Dallas*, p. 109.
13. House Select Committee on Assassinations Report, Vol. II, p. 63.

14. House Select Committee on Assassinations Report, Vol. VIII, p. 105.
15. House Select Committee on Assassinations Report, Vol. VI, p. 17.
16. Ibid.
17. Warren Commission Report, p. 612.
18. Sabato, Larry. *The Kennedy Half-Century: The Presidency, Assassination, and Lasting Legacy of John F. Kennedy*, pp. 241 – 248.
19. Thomas, Donald. *Hear No Evil*, p. 702.
20. Thomas, Donald. *Hear No Evil*, p. 561.
21. Thompson, Josiah. *Six Seconds in Dallas*, p. 25.
22. Nelson, Phillip. *LBJ: The Mastermind of the JFK Assassination*, p. 450.
23. Warren Commission Hearings and Exhibits, Vol. VI, p 205.
24. Interview of Jean Hill, FBI report by SA Robert C. Lish, Nov. 23, 1963, file no. DL 89-43.
25. Interview of Jean Hill, Mar. 17, 1964, FBI report by SA E.J. Robertson and Thomas T. Trettis, file no. DL 89-43, p. 2.
26. House Select Committee on Assassinations Report, Vol. XII, p. 10.
27. Warren Commission Hearings and Exhibits, Vol. VI, p. 207.
28. Marrs, Jim. *Crossfire: The Plot That Killed Kennedy*, p. 483.
29. Sullivan, William. *The Bureau*, p. 52.
30. Warren Commission Hearings and Exhibits, Vol. IV, p 133.
31. House Select Committee on Assassinations Report, Vol. IV, p. 147.

CHAPTER 8

1. New York Times, January 24, 2007, p. C13.
2. Hedegaard, Erik. *The Last Confessions of E. Howard Hunt*, Rolling Stone, April 5, 2007.
3. Ibid.
4. Ventura, Jesse, Russell, Dick, and Wayne, David. *They Killed Our President*, p. 261.
5. Nelson, Phillip. *LBJ: The Mastermind of the JFK Assassination*, p 82.
6. Corsi, Jerome. *Who Really Killed Kennedy?*, pp. 254, 291 – 294.
7. Waldron, Lamar, and Hartmann, Thom. *Ultimate Sacrifice*, pp. 506 – 508, 702 – 704.
8. O'Leary, Brad, and Seymour, L.E. *Triangle of Death: The Shocking*

Truth about the Role of South Vietnam and the French Mafia in the Assassination of JFK, pp. 58 – 97.

9. Hedegaard, Erik. *The Last Confessions of E. Howard Hunt*, Rolling Stone, April 5, 2007.
10. Ventura, Jesse. *Conspiracy Theory: JFK*, 35:00 – 42:00.
11. Groden, Robert, and Livingstone, Harrison. *High Treason: The Assassination of President Kennedy - What Really Happened*, p. 274.
12. Groden, Robert, and Livingstone, Harrison. *High Treason: The Assassination of President Kennedy - What Really Happened*, p. 142.
13. Hearings Before the Select Committee on Assassinations, Vol. 10, p. 172.
14. House Select Committee on Assassinations: Marita Lorenz Immunized Testimony, pp. 42 – 56, 122.
15. Marrs, Jim. *Crossfire: The Plot That Killed Kennedy*, p. 539.

CHAPTER 9

1. Marrs, Jim. Crossfire: *The Plot that Killed Kennedy*, p. 499.
2. Garrison, Jim. *On the Trail of the Assassins*, p. 103.
3. Thomas, Kenn, and Childress, David. *Nasa, Nazis and JFK*.
4. Thomas, Kenn, and Childress, David. *Nasa, Nazis and JFK,* pp. 195 – 197.
5. Farrell, Joseph. *LBJ and the Conspiracy to Kill Kennedy: A Coalescence of Interests*, p. 268.
6. Garrison, Jim. *On the Trail of the Assassins*, pp. 202, 222.
7. Thomas, Kenn, and Childress, David. *Nasa, Nazis and JFK,* p. 24.
8. Thomas, Kenn, and Childress, David. *Nasa, Nazis and JFK,* p. 29.
9. Thomas, Kenn, and Childress, David. *Nasa, Nazis and JFK,* p. 25.
10. Thomas, Kenn, and Childress, David. *Nasa, Nazis and JFK,* p. 28.
11. Thomas, Kenn, and Childress, David. *Nasa, Nazis and JFK,* p. 34.
12. Thomas, Kenn, and Childress, David. *Nasa, Nazis and JFK,* pp. 26 – 27.
13. Stone, Roger, and Colapietro, Mike. *The Man Who Killed Kennedy: The Case Against LBJ*, p. 334.
14. New York Times, November 10, 1977, p. 94.
15. Thomas, Kenn, and Childress, David. *Nasa, Nazis and JFK,* pp. 35, 52.

16. Thomas, Kenn, and Childress, David. *Nasa, Nazis and JFK,* pp. 48 - 49.
17. Thomas, Kenn, and Childress, David. *Nasa, Nazis and JFK,* pp. 74 – 76.
18. Thomas, Kenn, and Childress, David. *Nasa, Nazis and JFK,* pp. 76 – 77.
19. Thomas, Kenn, and Childress, David. *Nasa, Nazis and JFK,* p. 55.
20. Thomas, Kenn, and Childress, David. *Nasa, Nazis and JFK,* p. 71.
21. Reid, Ed, and Demaris, Ovid. *The Green Felt Jungle.*
22. Kennedy, Robert, *The Enemy Within.*
23. Thomas, Kenn, and Childress, David. *Nasa, Nazis and JFK,* pp. 71 – 72.
24. Reid, Ed. *The Grim Reapers.*
25. Thomas, Kenn, and Childress, David. *Nasa, Nazis and JFK,* p. 59.
26. Thomas, Kenn, and Childress, David. *Nasa, Nazis and JFK,* pp. 86 – 90.
27. Thomas, Kenn, and Childress, David. *Nasa, Nazis and JFK,* p. 117.
28. Garrison, Jim. *On the Trail of the Assassins*, p. 101.
29. Thomas, Kenn, and Childress, David. *Nasa, Nazis and JFK,* p. 103.
30. Warren Commission Report, p. 305.
31. Thomas, Kenn, and Childress, David. *Nasa, Nazis and JFK,* pp. 109 – 114.
32. Thomas, Kenn, and Childress, David. *Nasa, Nazis and JFK,* pp. 106 – 114.
33. Thomas, Kenn, and Childress, David. *Nasa, Nazis and JFK,* pp. 114 – 115.
34. Thomas, Kenn, and Childress, David. *Nasa, Nazis and JFK,* pp. 53, 126.
35. Thomas, Kenn, and Childress, David. *Nasa, Nazis and JFK,* p. 26.
36. Thomas, Kenn, and Childress, David. *Nasa, Nazis and JFK,* p. 40.
37. Garrison, Jim. *On the Trail of the Assassins*, Chapter 6.
38. Corsi, Jerome. *Who Really Killed JFK?*, pp. 301 – 315.

CHAPTER 10

1. Summers, Anthony. *Official and Confidential: The Secret Life of J. Edgar Hoover*, pp. 237 – 275.
2. Summers, Anthony. *Official and Confidential: The Secret Life of J. Edgar Hoover*, p. 49.
3. Summers, Anthony. *Official and Confidential: The Secret Life of J. Edgar Hoover*, p 94.

4. Summers, Anthony. *Official and Confidential: The Secret Life of J. Edgar Hoover*, p. 9.

5. Gentry, Curt, *J. Edgar Hoover: The Man and His Secrets*, p. 148.

6. Sullivan, William. *The Bureau*, p. 49.

7. White House tape transcripts, Oct. 8, 1971, cited in Summers, Anthony. *Official and Confidential: The Secret Life of J. Edgar Hoover*, p. 9.

8. Summers, Anthony. *Official and Confidential: The Secret Life of J. Edgar Hoover*, p. 47.

9. Summers, Anthony. *Official and Confidential: The Secret Life of J. Edgar Hoover*, p. 429.

10. Summers, Anthony. *Official and Confidential: The Secret Life of J. Edgar Hoover*, pp. 76 – 86.

11. Sullivan, William. *The Bureau*, p. 109.

12. Summers, Anthony. *Official and Confidential: The Secret Life of J. Edgar Hoover*, pp. 248 – 258.

13. Ibid.

14. Summers, Anthony. *Official and Confidential: The Secret Life of J. Edgar Hoover*, pp. 232 – 240.

15. Theoharis, Athan. *From the Secret Files of J. Edgar Hoover*, pp. 265, 284, 295.

16. Hack, Richard, *Puppetmaster: The Secret Life of J. Edgar Hoover*, p. 281.

17. Theoharis, Athan. *From the Secret Files of J. Edgar Hoover*, pp. 284 – 285.

18. Theoharis, Athan. *From the Secret Files of J. Edgar Hoover*, pp. 285 – 286.

19. Theoharis, Athan. *From the Secret Files of J. Edgar Hoover*, p. 286.

20. Theoharis, Athan, and Cox, Stuart, *The Boss: J. Edgar Hoover and the Great American Inquisition,* pp. 208 – 212.

21. Theoharis, Athan. *From the Secret Files of J. Edgar Hoover*, p. 4.

22. Summers, Anthony. *Official and Confidential: The Secret Life of J. Edgar Hoover*, p. 94.

23. Theoharis, Athan. *From the Secret Files of J. Edgar Hoover*, p. 15.

24. Theoharis, Athan. *From the Secret Files of J. Edgar Hoover*, pp. 24 – 25.

25. Marrs, Jim. *Crossfire: The Plot that Killed Kennedy*, p. 223.

26. Summers, Anthony. *Official and Confidential: The Secret Life of J.*

Edgar Hoover, p. 271.

27. Russell, Dick. *The Man Who Knew Too Much*, p. 54.

28. New York Times, November 25, 1963, p. 8.

29. Russell, Dick. *On the Trail of the Assassins – A Revealing Look at America's Most Infamous Unsolved Crime*, p. 452.

30. Russell, Dick. *The Man Who Knew Too Much*, pp. 53 - 59.

31. Nelson, Phillip. *LBJ: The Mastermind of the JFK Assassination*, pp. 362 – 363.

32. Powers, Richard. *Secrecy and Power: The Life of J. Edgar Hoover*, p. 353.

33. Giancana, Antoinette, Hughes, John, and Jobe, Thomas. *JFK and Sam: The Connection Between the Giancana and Kennedy Assassinations*, p. 88.

34. Sullivan, William. *The Bureau*, p. 48.

35. Nash, Jay. *Citizen Hoover*, p. 149.

36. Powers, Richard. *Secrecy and Power: The Life of J. Edgar Hoover*, p. 365.

CHAPTER 11

1. History Channel. *The Men Who Killed Kennedy: The Guilty Men*, 1:30 – 2:00.

2. History Channel. *The Men Who Killed Kennedy: The Guilty Men*, 3:30 – 5:30.

3. History Channel. *The Men Who Killed Kennedy: The Guilty Men*, 10:25 – 13:50.

4. History Channel. *The Men Who Killed Kennedy: The Guilty Men*, 2:20 – 3:30.

5. McClellan, Barr. *Blood, Money and Power*.

6. Beschloss, Michael. *Taking Charge: The Johnson White House Tapes, 1963 – 1964*. p. 321.

7. Summers, Anthony. *Official and Confidential: The Secret Life of J. Edgar Hoover*, p. 310.

8. Dallek, Robert. *Flawed Giant: Lyndon Johnson and His Times*, pp. 40 - 41.

9. Dallek, Robert. *Lyndon B. Johnson, Portrait of a President*, p. 140.
10. Henggeler, Paul. *Lyndon Johnson and the Kennedy Mystique*, p. 64.
11. Marrs, Jim. *Crossfire: The Plot That Killed Kennedy*, p. 298.
12. History Channel. *The Men Who Killed Kennedy: The Guilty Men*, 20:00 – 25:45.
13. Stone, Roger, and Colapietro, Mike. *The Man Who Killed Kennedy: The Case Against LBJ*, pp. 178 – 179.
14. Nelson, Phillip. *LBJ: The Mastermind of the JFK Assassination*, pp. 307-311.
15. Marrs, Jim. *Crossfire: The Plot That Killed Kennedy*, p. 297.
16. Stone, Roger, and Colapietro, Mike. *The Man Who Killed Kennedy: The Case Against LBJ*, pp. 252 – 253.
17. Zirbel, Craig. *The Texas Connection: The Assassination of John F. Kennedy*, pp. 18 – 21.
18. Marrs, Jim. *Crossfire: The Plot That Killed Kennedy*, p. 297.
19. Caro, Robert. *Master of the Senate*, pp. 121 – 122.
20. Kearns, Doris. *Lyndon Johnson and the American Dream*.
21. O'Reilly, Bill. *Killing Kennedy*, p. 91.
22. Dallek, Robert. *Flawed Giant: Lyndon Johnson and His Times 1961 – 1973*, p. 491.
23. Caro, Robert. *Master of the Senate*, pp. 121 – 122.
24. Gillon, Steven. *The Kennedy Assassination - 24 Hours After: Lyndon B. Johnson's Pivotal First Day as President*, p. 7.

CHAPTER 12

1. Dallek, Robert. *Lyndon B. Johnson: Portrait of a President*, p. 150.
2. Beschloss, Michael. *Reaching for Glory: Lyndon Johnson's Secret White House Tapes, 1964 – 1965*, p. 54.
3. Washington Post, November 24, 1963, p. A2.
4. History Channel. *LBJ vs The Kennedys: Chasing Demons*, 43:25 – 44:30.
5. Beschloss, Michael. *Reaching for Glory: Lyndon Johnson's Secret White House Tapes, 1964 – 1965*, p. 54.
6. Dallek, Robert. *Lyndon B. Johnson, Portrait of a President*, p. 188.

7. Washington Post, February 19, 2009.
8. Stone, Roger, and Colapietro, Mike. *The Man Who Killed Kennedy: The Case Against LBJ*, pp. 29 – 30.
9. Sullivan, William. *The Bureau*, p. 70.
10. Dallek, Robert, *Flawed Giant: Lyndon Johnson and His Times*, pp. 179 – 181.
11. Sullivan, William. *The Bureau*, p. 69.
12. Centers of Disease Control and Prevention, *Morbidity and Mortality Report*, Vol. 62, No. 7, p. 1.
13. New York Times, March 29, 1992, p. H23.
14. Garrison, Jim. *On the Trail of the Assassins*, pp. 273 – 274, 294, 323.
15. Warren Commission Report, p. 803.
16. Warren Commission Hearings and Exhibits, Vol. XIV, pp. 312 - 313.
17. Warren Commission Hearings and Exhibits, Commission Exhibit 2505, Vol. XXV, p. 716.
18. Warren Commission Hearings and Exhibits, Commission Exhibit 2398, Vol. XXV, p. 377.
19. Warren Commission Hearings and Exhibits, Commission Exhibit 2795, Vol. XXVI, pp. 184 – 185.
20. Warren Commission Hearings and Exhibits, Commission Exhibit 3013, Vol. XXVI, pp. 548 – 549.
21. Waldron, Lamar. *Legacy of Secrecy: The Long Shadow of the JFK Assassination*, p. 53.
22. O'Leary, Brad, and Seymour, L.E. *Triangle of Death: The Shocking Truth about the Role of South Vietnam and the French Mafia in the Assassination of JFK*, p. 179.
23. House Select Committee on Assassinations Report, Vol. 11, p. 291.
24. Las Vegas Review Journal, May 7, 2000, p. 3a.
25. Warren Commission Hearings and Exhibits, Vol. XIV, pp. 599 – 615.
26. House Select Committee on Assassinations Report, Vol. 3, p. 471.
27. Groden, Robert. *The Search for Lee Harvey Oswald*, p. 31.
28. Warren Commission Hearings and Exhibits, Vol. XI, pp. 325 – 339.
29. New Orleans Grand Jury Proceedings, March 16, 1967, pp. 22 – 23.
30. Kurtz, Michael. *The JFK Assassination Debates*, p. 164.
31. Groden, Robert. *The Search for Lee Harvey Oswald*, pp. 20 – 21.
32. Groden, Robert. *The Search for Lee Harvey Oswald*, p. 28.
33. Ventura, Jesse, Russell, Dick, and Wayne, David. *They Killed Our*

President, pp. 300 – 301.

34. O'Reilly, Bill, and Dugard, Martin. *Killing Kennedy: The End of Camelot*, p. 103.

35. Phelan, James. *Scandals, Scamps, and Scoundrels*, pp. 150 – 151.

36. Warren Commission Report, p. 661.

37. Warren Commission Report, p. 662.

38. Warren Commission Report, p. 650.

39. Warren Commission Hearings and Exhibits, Vol. I, p. 238.

40. Garrison, Jim. *On the Trail of the Assassins*, p. 252.

41. History Channel. *JFK: 3 Shots That Changed America*, 1:35:00 – 1:36:35.

42. History Channel. *The Men Who Killed Kennedy: The Witnesses*, 20:45 – 22:30.

43. Stone, Roger, and Colapietro, Mike. *The Man Who Killed Kennedy: The Case Against LBJ*, p. 186.

44. Nelson, Phillip. *LBJ: The Mastermind of the JFK Assassination*, p. 184.

45. Stone, Roger, and Colapietro, Mike. *The Man Who Killed Kennedy: The Case Against LBJ*, p. 290.

46. Warren Commission Hearings and Exhibits, Commission Exhibit 343, Vol. XVI, p. 942.

47. Warren Commission Report, p.158.

CHAPTER 13

1. Lane, Mark. *Plausible Denial: Was the CIA Involved in the Assassination of JFK?*, p. 131.

2. Davis, John. *Mafia Kingfish: Carlos Marcello and the Assassination of John F. Kennedy*, p. 135.

3. Garrison, Jim. *On the Trail of the Assassins*, pp. 356 – 357.

4. O'Leary, Brad, and Seymour, L.E. *Triangle of Death: The Shocking Truth about the Role of South Vietnam and the French Mafia in the Assassination of JFK*, p. 203.

5. Warren Commission Report, pp. 14 – 15.

CHAPTER 14

1. Nelson, Phillip. *LBJ: The Mastermind of the JFK Assassination*, p. 320.
2. O'Leary, Brad, and Seymour, L.E. *Triangle of Death: The Shocking Truth about the Role of South Vietnam and the French Mafia in the Assassination of JFK*, pp. 172 – 181, p. 203.

BIBLIOGRAPHY

Beschloss, Michael. *Reaching for Glory: Lyndon Johnson's Secret White House Tapes, 1964 – 1965*. New York: Simon and Schuster, 2001.

Beschloss, Michael. *Taking Charge: The Johnson White House Tapes, 1963 – 1964*. New York: Simon and Schuster, 1997.

Blakey, G. Robert, and Billings, Richard. *The Plot to Kill the President: Organized Crime Assassinated JFK*. New York: Times Books, 1981.

Bugliosi, Vincent. *Reclaiming History*. New York: Norton, 2007.

Caro, Robert. *The Master of the Senate*. New York: Knopf, 2002.

Childs, Allen. *We Were There: Revelations from the Dallas Doctors Who Attended to JFK on November 22, 1963*. New York: Skyhorse Publishing, 2013.

Corsi, Jerome. *Who Really Killed Kennedy?* Washington: WND Books, 2013.

Corson, William, Trento, Susan, and Trento, Joseph. *Widows*. New York: MacDonald, 1989.

Dallek, Robert. *Flawed Giant: Lyndon Johnson and His Times*. New York: Oxford University Press, 1998.

Dallek, Robert. *Lyndon B. Johnson, Portrait of a President*. New York: Oxford University Press, 2004.

Davis, John. *Mafia Kingfish: Carlos Marcello and the Assassination of John F. Kennedy*. New York: McGraw-Hill, 1988.

Elliott, Todd. *A Rose By Many Other Names: Rose Cherami and the JFK Assassination*. Walterville, Oregon: Trine Day, 2013.

Epstein, Edward Jay. *Inquest: The Warren Commission and the Establishment of Truth*. New York: Viking Press, 1966.

Farrell, Joseph. *LBJ and the Conspiracy to Kill Kennedy: A Coalescence of Interests*. Kempton, Illinois: Adventures Unlimited, 2011.

Garrison, Jim. *On the Trail of the Assassins*. New York: Warner, 1988.

Gentry, Curt. *J. Edgar Hoover: The Man and His Secrets*. New York: Penguin, 1992.

Gillon, Steven. *The Kennedy Assassination - 24 Hours After: Lyndon B. Johnson's Pivotal First Day as President*. New York: Basic Books; 2010.

Giancana, Antoinette, Hughes, John, and Jobe, Thomas. *JFK and Sam: The Connection Between the Giancana and Kennedy Assassinations*. Nashville: Cumberland House, 2005.

Groden, Robert. *The Search for Lee Harvey Oswald*. New York: Penguin, 1995.

Groden, Robert, and Livingstone, Harrison. *High Treason: The Assassination of President Kennedy - What Really Happened*. New York: Berkley, 1989.

Hack, Richard, *Puppetmaster: The Secret Life of J. Edgar Hoover*. Beverly Hills: New Millenium, 2004.

Henggeler, Paul. *In His Steps: Lyndon Johnson and the Kennedy Mystique*. Chicago: Ivan Dee, 1991.

History Channel. *JFK: 3 Shots That Changed America.* A&E Television Networks, 2009.

History Channel. *LBJ vs The Kennedys: Chasing Demons*.

History Channel. *The Men Who Killed Kennedy: The Guilty Men*.

History Channel. *The Men Who Killed Kennedy: The Truth Shall Set You Free*.

Hougan, Jim. *Secret Agenda*. New York: Random House, 1984.

Janney, Peter. *Mary's Mosaic*. New York: Skyhorse Publishing, 2012.

Kearns, Doris. *Lyndon Johnson and the American Dream*. New York: St. Martin's Press, 1991.

Kennedy, Robert, *The Enemy Within*. New York: Harper and Row, 1960.

Kurtz, Michael. *The JFK Assassination Debates*. Kansas: University Press, 2006.

Lane, Mark. *Rush to Judgment*. New York: Holt, Rinehart, and Winston, 1966.

Lane, Mark. *Plausible Denial: Was the CIA Involved in the Assassination of JFK?* New York: Thunder's Mouth Press, 1991.

Lattimer, John. *Kennedy and Lincoln: Medical and Ballistic Comparisons of Their Assassinations*. New York: Harcourt Brace Jovanovich, 1980.

Lifton, David S. *Best Evidence: Disguise and Deception in the Assassination of John F. Kennedy*. New York: Macmillan, 1980.

Livingstone, Harrison. *High Treason 2, The Great Coverup: The Assassination of President John F. Kennedy*. New York: Carroll and Graf, 1992.

Marrs, Jim. Crossfire: *The Plot that Killed Kennedy*, New York: Carroll and

Graf, 1989.

McClellan, Barr. *Blood, Money and Power – How LBJ Killed JFK.* New York: Hannover House, 2003.

Nash, Jay. *Citizen Hoover*. Chicago: Nelson-Hall, 1972.

Nelson, Phillip. *LBJ: The Mastermind of the JFK Assassination*. New York: Skyhorse Publishing, 2011.

O'Leary, Brad, and Seymour, L.E. *Triangle of Death: The Shocking Truth about the Role of South Vietnam and the French Mafia in the Assassination of JFK.* Nashville: WND Books, 2003.

O'Reilly, Bill, and Dugard, Martin. *Killing Kennedy: The End of Camelot.* New York: Holt, 2012.

Phelan, James. *Scandals, Scamps, and Scoundrels*. New York: Random House, 1982.

Posner, Gerald. *Case Closed: Lee Harvey Oswald and the Assassination of JFK.* New York: Random House, 1993.

Powers, Richard. *Secrecy and Power: The Life of J. Edgar Hoover*. New York: Macmillan, 1987.

Reid, Ed. *The Grim Reapers.* Chicago: Regnery, 1969.

Reid, Ed, and Demaris, Ovid. *The Green Felt Jungle*. New York: Trident, 1963.

Report of the President's Commission on the Assassination of President John F. Kennedy. Washington: U.S. Government Printing Office, 1964 (reprinted by Longmeadow Press, Stamford, Connecticut, 1993).

Report of the Select Committee on Assassinations, U.S. House of Representatives. Washington: U.S. Government Printing Office, 1979.

Russell, Dick. *The Man Who Knew Too Much*, New York: Carroll and Graf, 1992.

Sabato, Larry. *The Kennedy Half-Century: The Presidency, Assassination, and Lasting Legacy of John F. Kennedy*. New York: Bloomsbury, 2013.

Stone, Roger, and Colapietro, Mike. *The Man Who Killed Kennedy: The Case Against LBJ.* New York: Skyhorse Publishing, 2013.

Sullivan, William. *The Bureau*. New York: Norton, 1979.

Summers, Anthony. *Official and Confidential: The Secret Life of J. Edgar Hoover*. New York: Putnam, 1993.

Summers, Anthony. *Not in Your Lifetime*, New York: Open Road, 2013.

Theoharis, Athan. *From the Secret Files of J. Edgar Hoover*. Chicago: Ivan Dee, 1991.

Theoharis, Athan, and Cox, Stuart, *The Boss: J. Edgar Hoover and the Great American Inquisition*. Philadelphia: Temple University Press, 1988.

Thomas, Donald. *Hear No Evil: Politics, Science & the Forensic Evidence in the Kennedy Assassination*. New York: Skyhorse Publishing, 2010.

Thomas, Kenn, and Childress, David. *Nasa, Nazis and JFK*. Kempton, Illinois: Adventures Unlimited Press, 1996.

Thompson, Josiah. *Six Seconds in Dallas*. New York: Random House, 1967.

Ventura, Jesse. *Conspiracy Theory: JFK*, 35:00 – 42:00.

Ventura, Jesse, Russell, Dick, and Wayne, David. *They Killed Our President*. New York: Skyhorse Publishing, 2013.

Waldron, Lamar, and Hartmann, Thom. *Ultimate Sacrifice*. Berkeley: Counterpoint, 2009.

Weisberg, Harold. *John F. Kennedy Post Mortem*. Harold Weisberg, Publisher, 1975.

Zirbel, Craig. *The Texas Connection: The Assassination of John F. Kennedy*. Scottsdale, Arizona: The Texas Connection Company, 1991.

CREDITS

1. Figure 1-1: Corbis.

2. Figures 1-5, 3-5, 7-3, 7-8, 7-9, and 7-11: Zapruder Film © 1967 (Renewed 1995), The Sixth Floor Museum at Dealey Plaza.

3. Figure 3-4: Getty Images.

4. Figure 5-7: Corbis.

5. Figure 7-2: Malcolm E. Barker Collection / The Sixth Floor Museum at Dealey Plaza.

6. Figure 7-6: Corbis.

INDEX

257

43 ~~████~~ DICS for Gov. Connolly

ABOUT THE AUTHOR

The author holds a neuroscience doctorate. He is a former university and adjunct medical school professor, and has also worked extensively in industry and government.

Page 121
122
156 EVIL DOERS ⊗
154 OZZIE, OZZIE

49 Gov DRS.
48